7 MAY 2025

KV-072-746

AWN

Library and orr
alvor eeaby

Foundations of health care

Ethical dilemmas and communicative challenges

YORK ST. JOHN
COLLEGE LIBRARY

Unipub 2009

York St John

3 8025 00553182 0

©Unipub 2009

ISBN 978-82-7477-447-6

Contact info Unipub:
T: + 47 22 85 33 00
F: + 47 22 85 30 39
E-mail: post@unipub.no
www.unipub.no

Publisher: Oslo Academic Press, Unipub Norway
Design and layout: Oslo Academic Press, Unipub Norway
Printed in Norway: AIT e-dit AS

Printed with the support from the University College in Lillehammer

All rights reserved. No part of this publication may be reproduced or
transmitted, in any form or by any means, without permission

Contents

Chapter 7

Preface

This book addresses ethical dilemmas and communicative challenges in medicine and health care from a philosophical perspective. Four of the chapters have been previously published as articles; three (the first, sixth and seventh) are new to this book.

The reasons for this collection are twofold. The first is practical. As the articles have originally been published in different journals, I have wanted to bring them together into one publication. My idea is that this book can be useful both as a source for researchers who are interested in the philosophy of medicine and health care and as core literature for higher-level courses that focus on the fundamental issues of understanding and ethics involved in health personnel-patient interaction. Secondly, all the chapters relate to each other thematically. Although it would be too much to say that they jointly express a general philosophical system, there are many common themes and argumentative perspectives. One important consequence of this interconnectedness is that a good understanding of the arguments of one chapter is easer to acquire if they are interpreted in the light of the other chapters.

The first chapter attempts to explain the nature of my general philosophical approach. This chapter aims to clarify the fruitfulness both of a philosophical approach to issues of understanding and ethics in health care and of my perspective in particular. In my opinion, philosophy is too often regarded as a pure, abstract subject that cannot shed any useful and practical light on real-life problems and challenges. As in other areas, this sceptical view has sometimes been expressed in medicine and health care. This is a view I am strongly opposed to, and an important aim of this book is to show that it is unjustified. In this sense I hope I can be an ambassador not only for philosophy, but also for the more general idea that the best solutions to real-life communicative challenges and ethical dilemmas are theory-based. Scepticism about applied philosophy often has its source in a more fundamental scepticism about the practical usefulness of abstract theories and in a corresponding enthusiastic embracing of a very dualistic theory-practice distinction. In my view, this scepticism and dogmatic faith in a sharp distinction between theory and practice are fundamentally unjustified. The main reason is that ethical or communicative action-guiding principles, rules or procedures do not have a determinate normative content unless they are understood in the light of a theoretical framework that clarifies the central concepts.

Consider as an example the vague moral principle that 'All patients should be treated with appropriate respect'. This sentence strikes us as true, but that is because it is almost a platitude. Everyone thinks that patients should be treated with appropriate respect, given such practical limits as the time one has to offer care and so on. The point is that the sentence does not in itself say anything about what it is to treat a patient with due respect – it is unclear which actions would be recommended as 'good' and which would be 'bad'. The clarification of such distinctions is the job of an underlying theory. We need a theory that explains what it is to treat a patient with appropriate respect, so that it is easier to determine whether or not specific actions correspond to this moral principle.

The problem is that, nowadays, students are not always interested in studying abstract theories that do not have any immediate practical consequences. Students often want to learn something that they can understand right away, a 'list of principles' clearly linked to their existing or future health-care practices, almost like recipes for securing successful communication and good solutions to ethical problems. But here is the rub: the easier it is to learn a simple 'theory' with immediate practical consequences, the less the theory will have any real, substantial implications. In my view, any *significant* theory about communication or ethics in health care *must* be rather abstract – and thereby often challenging to learn and understand for students without philosophical training – if it is going to shed any interesting light on real-life challenges and dilemmas.

Obviously, this does not mean that a philosophical theory about communication or ethics necessarily has plausible implications. In order for a set of implications to be plausible, it is not *sufficient* that they are based on a theory; it is also *necessary* that this theory be based on convincing arguments. I do not claim, then, that the arguments in this book necessarily give 'correct' solutions to the problems I focus on simply because the answers are grounded on robust theoretical frameworks. The reader needs to study critically these theoretical frameworks and the arguments I have presented in favour of them in order to form his own ideas about the plausibility of the theories and the soundness of their implications.

Many people have helped me to develop the arguments in this book, and I would like to thank all of them. I am especially indebted to the anonymous referee who has read the three new chapters and has generously offered useful comments. Truls Petersen in the publishing company has been of invaluable assistance in taking care of many practical aspects of this project. I would not have been able to finish the book without the excellent cooperation with him and Unipub. I would also like to thank the University College in Lillehammer for funding this undertaking. And last, but not least, I cannot fully express my gratitude for Cecilie, Sigurd, and Marie for their great support from home!

Chapters previously published

- 'Meaning and normativity in nurse-patient-interaction' was originally published in *Nursing Philosophy*, 1, 2007.

- 'Interactive and face-to-face communication: a perspective from philosophy of mind and language' was originally published in *Seminar.net*, 3, 2006.
- 'The analytic-synthetic distinction and conceptual analyses of basic health concepts' was originally published in *Medicine, Health Care and Philosophy*, 2, 2006.
- 'Wittgenstein's theory of conceptual competence and virtue analyses of ethical dilemmas in nursing practice' was originally published in *Online Journal of Health Ethics*, 1, 2008.

Chapter 1

Communication and ethics in medicine and health care: the significance of a philosophical approach

1. Introduction

This book focuses on communicative challenges and ethical dilemmas within the field of medicine and health care. What the arguments and analyses have in common is that they are based on philosophical theories and not directly on empirical investigations. The discussions refer to empirical research, but this is research that has already been done and documented in existing literature. In this sense the book belongs within what is often called 'meta-analysis' and sometimes 'studies of literature'. However, a more suitable and informative label is 'applied philosophy' (Grayling 1998): all the chapters address fundamental problems and challenges in patient interaction on the basis of central assumptions in modern moral philosophy and philosophy of language. This applied approach is the core and central part of the defined area *philosophy of medicine and health care* (Wulff 1992; Nordenfelt 2001).

People sometimes ask me about the usefulness of a philosophical discussion that does not offer us any new interesting empirical facts: 'Are not discussions on communication and ethics rather pointless without making your own investigations?' My immediate answer is that this question presupposes a very narrow idea both of what science is and of how science can help us to address fundamental questions that affect us all (Hollis 1994; Chalmers 2005). This answer is, admittedly, one that requires further justification, and this book can be understood as an attempt to show how philosophy, even as a rather abstract discipline, can shed important light on central issues related to communication and ethics in health care. None of the chapters below, however, says anything general about the significance of a philosophical approach in this area. In order to understand fully the practical relevance of the book, I therefore think it is important to clarify some of the most important conceptual relations between philosophy and health care, and this is the task of this initial chapter.

2. Bottom-up and top-down methodology

On the most general level, we can explain the crucial difference between an empirical and a philosophical approach to communication and ethics by using the distinction between a 'bottom-up' and a 'top-down' methodological strategy (Hollis 1994; Chalmers 2005).

A bottom-up strategy will make empirical investigations, by using qualitative or quantitative methods, and then seek to derive conclusions from these investigations. The overall aim is to capture observable facts or 'data' and then to establish reasonable, scientific conclusions on the basis of these facts (Chalmers 2005). The more empirical the approach is, the less will it allow conclusions to capture more than what is strictly speaking 'contained in the facts'. Bottom-up strategies are typically used in the natural sciences such as biology, archaeology, geology, and in many parts of medicine (Hollis 1994).

Bottom-up approaches differ depending on the theoretical assumptions on which the empirical investigations are based. Grounded theory seeks to use as few theoretical assumptions as possible – everything should be built up from pure, theory-neutral observation (Glaser and Strauss 1967). The opposite approach is a rich interpretational hermeneutics that seeks to uncover underlying or 'hidden' meaning – such an approach might even presuppose that informers do not mean what they, strictly speaking, *say* in research interviews (Flick 2002; Gubrium and Holstein 2002). The more abstract and controversial the theoretical frameworks that are used to interpret informers are, the more likely it is that some will question the scientific validity of the conclusions of the research.

Although qualitative method falls under bottom-up approaches, it is generally acknowledged that it is impossible to conduct interviews without making *any* theoretical assumptions (Gubrium and Holstein 2002). Interpretation of informers will always be shaped by inter-viewers' personal horizons, knowledge of the area of discourse, and assumptions about the nature of poor and successful communication (Dahlberg, Drew and Nyström 2001). Thus, although conclusions in qualitative research are based on interviews or participant-observations, there is always a top-down dimension as well. This fact partly explains why some have been sceptical of the claim that qualitative method is properly scientific.

In contrast to a pure bottom-up strategy or a hybrid qualitative approach, a pure top-down strategy will not make any empirical investigations. It will instead focus on a theory and then discuss the implications of that theory within a given field of interest. Top-down strategies are often used in disciplines such as sociology, studies of literature, and last, but not least, in applied philosophy. In its most formal mode, a methodological top-down strategy uses nothing more than logical method: strict rules of logic become the only valid rules of inference that can be used to derive implications from a set of theoretical assumptions (Peacocke 1992; Grayling 1998).

This narrow logical approach offers few possibilities for deriving substantial implications from a philosophical theory; that is, it becomes very difficult to shed light on any real problems and challenges within the area one aims to analyse. Usually, a top-down approach will therefore allow for a wider concept of implication. The idea will be to derive reasonable implications, whereby 'reasonable' is understood in a broader sense that is not restricted to logical rationality (Peacocke

1992; Grayling 1998). All the arguments in this book belong within this wider approach.

3. A philosophical approach

The distinction between a methodological top-down and a bottom-up strategy is entirely general. As noted, we can find elements of this distinction in many different disciplines, but the distinction becomes especially salient if we compare the natural sciences with influential traditions within the humanities and social sciences.

What does it mean more specifically when a top-down strategy is philosophical? In other words, what are the special characteristics of applied philosophy? Philosophical approaches will differ depending on the nature of the philosophical theory and the area of interest, but there are two typical elements.

Most notably, an applied philosophy will seek to shed light on the area it aims to analyse. It will do this in three ways. First, the philosophical analysis will typically seek to clarify complex and often controversial concepts (Grayling 1998; Nordenfelt 2001). Indeed, this has sometimes been regarded as the main aim of philosophy of medicine and health care. Wulff writes, 'the core issue [of philosophy of medicine] is [...] the analysis of health and illness – the two concepts that define medical activities' (Wulff 1992, 85). Other central and disputed health concepts are *disease* and *sickness*, and in bioethics *patient autonomy, informed consent, empathy* and *care*. All of these concepts are discussed in this book.

Secondly, a philosophical approach will seek to clarify problems and challenges. Consider the idea of an ethical dilemma. Why is an ethical dilemma experienced as a dilemma? Why is it sometimes difficult to determine what a 'good' course of action is? As explained in the chapters on ethics below, if an encounter with a patient represents a genuine ethical dilemma for a health worker, then there must be some good reasons that weigh in favour of (at least) two alternative actions towards the patient (Davis et al. 1997). A philosophical discussion will seek to uncover these reasons, and thereby help to clarify why the dilemma is *felt* to be a dilemma from the perspective of the health worker. Any attempt to solve the ethical dilemma must show that one set of reasons outweighs the other(s). A philosophical approach with normative ambitions will characteristically seek to give health workers 'conceptual tools' for identifying the best set of reasons (Kushner and Thomasma 2001; Ashcroft et al. 2005).

The same point applies in analyses of communicative challenges. It is of fundamental importance for health workers to understand how and why it is important to secure successful communication with patients (Silverman et al. 2004). The probability of avoiding misunderstandings and poor communication is significantly reduced if health workers have some knowledge of how communicative challenges can be met. A philosophical analysis of communicative challenges in medicine and health care will attempt to give health workers this kind of practical knowledge (Ashcroft et al. 2005).

The result might be that a simple problem becomes more complex than what it seemed at first glance, but a complex problem might also become less complicated. As an example of the first kind of problem, consider situations in which doctors wonder whether it is correct to communicate the complete truth to patients (Gillon 2001; Higgs 2006), a situation which is discussed in the sixth chapter of this book. This question might seem straightforward, but, as I argue, it becomes more complex when one asks what it means to tell the truth to a patient. By clarifying what it is to be telling the truth in general, a philosophical analysis of truth-telling will attempt to make it easier for doctors to understand whether or not they have been engaged in truth-telling in specific cases.

To help clarify those problems that can become less complicated when they are subject to philosophical scrutiny, we can take as an example pre-hospital situations involving patients who do not wish to receive treatment and transport even though their symptoms indicate that they have a serious disease or injury (Sanders 2001). As explained in the seventh chapter below, medical paramedics attending these patients often confront the following dilemma: should they act in accordance with the patient's wishes or should they act paternalistically and let the patient be forced to receive necessary treatment and transport?

These alternatives might strike paramedics as the only genuine alternatives, but there is often a third way out of the problem. Sometimes patients will change their mind if they receive, in a very direct way, neutral and objective information about their state of health and the gravity of the situation. In that case, good communication has 'dissolved' the ethical dilemma; the patients change their preferences simply by understanding new factual information. An emphasis on the systematic analysis of ethical dilemmas – especially opening with clear communication of relevant factual knowledge of the conditions of disease or injury to the patient – is a key aspect of a philosophical analysis of communication and ethics in health care.

The third way an applied philosophy will clarify a field of interest is by evaluating ideological assumptions. This kind of examination involves more than clarifying concepts and straightforward assumptions that form the basis of a characterisation or an experience of a problem. The next ideological step involves a critical discussion of the assumptions that have been uncovered (Habermas 1984). The organisation of a medical practice is often shaped by an underlying scientific ideology, and a critical philosophy will often seek to uncover and challenge such ideologies (Yamada et al. 2008). An evidence-based medical practice will, for instance, have its source in positivist traditions within philosophy of science to a large extent.

A practice that instead emphasises the importance of 'soft' concepts like *empathy*, *care*, and *understanding* – concepts that cannot be measured in a straightforward way – are closely associated with the humanities and social sciences, and these practices are often believed to be incompatible with evidence-based approaches (Crawford et al. 1998). Philosophical analyses will often seek to identify and discuss critically such opposing ideologies by tracing them to more fundamental tensions between different scientific paradigms (Kuhn 1970; Hollis 1994; Nordenfelt 2001).

This ideological dimension is particularly striking within ethics. Many ethical practices in health care are heavily influenced by ethical ideologies. The most obvious tension is between a consequence-based approach that holds that health personnel should choose actions that have the 'best' consequences for patients, and a Kantian 'duty' approach that insists that health personnel should act in accordance with patients' own autonomous wishes (Kuhse and Singer 2001). As explained in the chapters on ethics in this book, these two ethical perspectives have strikingly different practical implications. Therefore, in the final instance, the course of actions towards a patient depends on which ethical perspective health workers find most plausible. But the evaluation of different ethical perspective is a philosophical project. As long as health workers have to *act* on the basis of ethical judgements, they have no choice but to engage in philosophical reasoning about the nature of 'good' actions.

4. The area of interest

The other central dimension of an applied top-down philosophical approach is that it has to be properly linked to the area it purports to analyse. In order to clarify the implications of a philosophical theory, it is insufficient to point out some vague and general consequences. Anyone who has taught students in health-care courses knows that a general knowledge of ethics and communication theory is pretty much useless if it is not connected to real-life examples and challenges. The students do not have a philosophical background, and they need help in relating philosophical analyses to their existing or future health-care practices. Indeed, nothing is as welcome as a good example that can clarify the consequences of a theory (Ashcroft et al. 2005).

There is at the same time a risk that an analysis can become too narrow (Davis et al. 1997). Resorting too extensively to particular examples can make it difficult for students to broaden their horizons. Students like down-to-earth case studies, and that is understandable, but sometimes insights into particular cases have limited value for generalisation. If a philosophical analysis merely focuses on one or a very few idiosyncratic cases, the conclusions might become too specific. It is important that students achieve a holistic understanding; they need to be able to understand how conclusions about particular cases apply in a variety of cases that are more or less similar (Ashcroft et al. 2005).

It should also be mentioned that within philosophy, examples are not used to justify but to clarify (Grayling 1998). The aim is not to use examples to validate a theory, but to show that the theory has substantial implications. The reason the examples should not be used to justify the theory is obvious: when a theorist in a philosophical discussion uses a few examples – they might even be examples that he has himself constructed – then the reader does not have a guarantee that the examples are representative. Showing that the examples are representative requires further empirical arguments, but developing such arguments is not a part of the applied philosophical project. For a philosopher, the crucial arguments are those he employs for his philosophical theory, but these arguments should be distinguished from the applied dimension of the theory.

This distinction does not imply that a philosophical theory is wholly divorced from the relevant data. It is not correct that philosophers always live in their own 'abstract world', detached from empirical facts and the empirical sciences. In fact, many assumptions in a philosophical theory might be justified empirically (Dancy 1991; Haack 1995). Consider, for instance, the idea of communication as involving the exchange of beliefs. The second chapter in this book explains how we have a fundamental belief that health workers often manage to communicate their own beliefs to patients, and that patients often manage to communicate their beliefs to health workers. This is something a philosopher typically will conceive of as an empirical fact, or at least an empirical contention that has a strong immediate appeal. Consequently, he will think that his philosophical theory about communication should incorporate this assumption. The theory should not imply that health workers and patients are very seldom able to share and communicate beliefs.

Similarly, a philosophical approach can be falsified empirically even though it is not a bottom-up strategy in the sense explained above. A philosophical theory aims to be consistent with plausible empirical theories. This means that if an empirical theory on which a philosophical analysis is based were to be weakened, then the philo-sophical theory would be weakened as well (Hollis 1994; Chalmers 2005). Sometimes a weakening of the empirical basis will affect the philosophical theory very directly. For example, if the abovementioned empirical contention that health workers and patients usually manage to communicate for some reason turns out to be implausible despite its immediate appeal, then a philosophical theory that is based on this assumption becomes implausible for the same reason.

5. Descriptive and normative dimensions

I have so far characterised an applied philosophical perspective by focusing on two aspects: the notion of critical clarification and the need to connect the philosophical implications to the area of analysis. There is another dimension that becomes especially salient within a health care context when the focus is on communication and ethics. A philosophical approach will typically be *normative*. The idea is simple enough. A pure empirical approach does not *evaluate* actions. A philosophical perspective, on the other hand, is normally action-guiding in the sense that it will claim that some actions are 'good' or 'correct' (Brink 1989).

This characteristic is most salient within ethics. The normative dimensions of ethical reflection have their own philosophical labels, 'normative ethics' and 'meta-ethics' (Brink 1989; Grayling 1998). Whereas theories within normative ethics seek to develop action-guiding norms, rules or principles, those within meta-ethics seek to justify normative theories, that is, the aim is to show why a given normative theory is plausible (Brink 1989; Dancy 2004). A purely empirical approach to ethics will be on a third level that is often called 'descriptive ethics'. Here the aim is to uncover and clarify the moral beliefs people actually have, without arguing for or against these beliefs (Brink 1989).

It is not often recognised that the same distinction between normative and descriptive approaches is also applicable to analyses of communication. Determining whether or not communication is successful cannot be done purely on the basis of empirical observations. It is also necessary to make theoretical 'meta' assumptions about the nature of poor and successful communication (Sperber and Wilson 1991). Furthermore, such assumptions have traditionally focused on the distinction between the 'inner' and 'outer'. The traditional idea has been that communication is successful if a sender manages to communicate a message he has in his 'inside his head' to the consciousness of an audience. But as explained in the third chapter below, this process cannot be observed in a straightforward way. Assumptions about communication, and especially the idea about a message that reaches the consciousness of an audience, are very much theoretical.

This does not mean that empirical facts cannot be part of a normative theory. The point is that empirical facts have to be combined with evaluative assumptions in order to be action-guiding. All too often theorists proceed too quickly from knowledge of empirical facts to what they think are substantial normative implications. This step requires independent arguments, and these arguments should always be clarified and defended. Many researchers are well aware of this, and the policy of many medical journals with an empirical focus is to exclude extensive normative discussions because they assume that such discussions call for further arguments and a different explanatory framework. It is a widespread view that it is better to let the empirical material speak for itself, and to let the readers reflect on the normative implications.

It is not difficult to understand why many medical journals have this policy, but sometimes one wishes that empirical analyses be less modest. Philosophers will often think that empirical facts about communication and ethics have immediate and interesting normative implications. Consider, for instance, empirical analyses that measure the quality of doctor-patient communication with respect to patient satisfaction (Silverman et al. 2004). If empirical investigations have revealed that a group of patients are not satisfied with doctors' communication, then a philosopher with normative ambitions will typically ask what the doctors should do in order to make the patients more satisfied. Within the practical limits of the relevant patient encounters, how can 'good' communicative actions contribute to achieve patient satisfaction?

More fundamentally, a philosopher is also likely to address critically the assumption that successful communication can be measured in terms of patient satisfaction. Is it always the case that a doctor has secured good communication if the patient is satisfied with the doctor's communication? What if the patient is satisfied simply because the doctor has given him a very positive prognosis? (We could even imagine that the prognosis is too optimistic and that the doctor has not communicated the truth.) Philosophers will typically emphasise that the assumption about patient satisfaction as sufficient for good communication is far from self-evident, and that it therefore needs to be justified.

The point about justification should be mentioned as an independent point. The concept of *justification* is one of the most central concepts within the philosophical discipline of epistemology – the study of the nature of belief and knowledge. Philosophers have traditionally asked what justification is, and how justification (together with true belief) can be sufficient for knowledge. A central issue concerns the question of regress (Dancy 1991; Haack 1995). When challenged to justify our beliefs, we typically appeal to other beliefs we harbour. But how can we know that these other beliefs are justified? We might yet again appeal to other beliefs, but the question stubbornly resurfaces: how is it possible to know that these beliefs are justified? Though these might strike us as rhetorical questions, a mere play with words, the adoption of a critical attitude is often valuable. Philosophers remind us that we should have beliefs that are as well justified as possible. In fact, even when we think that a belief is self-evident and does not require any further justification, then this is precisely a view that needs a justification. We should aim to be able to explain why the belief is self-evident (Wittgenstein 1969).

For the same reason a sceptical attitude may challenge us to explain why we think we know something about the world. Some famous philosophers like Descartes have endorsed general philosophical scepticism, the view that we do not know anything about the external world around us (Nordby 2009). However, scepticism might also be local within an area of discourse, like medicine and health care. Scepticism about doctor-patient communication is the view that doctors and patients are very seldom able to communicate (Nordby 2008a). Another sceptical view, discussed in the sixth chapter below, is that doctors are rarely able to communicate the whole truth about medical knowledge to patients who are laypeople (Henderson 1935). As long as we do not want to accept these sceptical conclusions, they force us to explain why the underlying arguments are implausible, that is, why doctors and patients manage to communicate and why doctors often manage to communicate the truth.

6. Communication and ethics

I have so far clarified the nature of applied philosophy, and I have, in particular, explained how philosophy can help us to elucidate important issues related to communication and ethics within medicine and health care. Obviously, the points I have made are quite abstract, and a more detailed explanation would require a more thorough analysis. The best suggestion I can give to those who are interested in achieving a better understanding the nature of philosophy of medicine and health care is to focus directly on specific discussions.

All of the chapters below are attempts to explain in more detail how philosophy can shed light on communicative challenges and ethical dilemmas in medicine and health care. In order to understand the specific philosophical arguments, the reader must study each chapter. Generally, the first three chapters focus on communication and the last three on ethics. Why then collect them into one book?

The reason is that I do not make a sharp distinction between communication and ethics. In fact, a main aim of the book is to show that communication and ethics should not be thought of as two different disciplines without any substantial connections.

In order to explain why this is so, I think it is fruitful to make a distinction between ethical challenges that arise within a communicative framework and communicative challenges that arise within an ethical framework. A good example of the former can be found in the third chapter in this book. Here I develop and discuss communication conditions, or conditions for successful patient communication. Now, one of these conditions focuses on values. Our personal values underlie many of our communicative actions, and they are crucial for understanding how we make ethical judgements (Raz 2005; Nordby 2008b). When we ascribe values like 'good' or 'bad' to actions – when we say things like 'That was a good action' – our intention is to communicate our value preferences to an audience. Successful communication presupposes that the audience understands what these value preferences are. If our audience misunderstands the values we express – if we are ascribed values that are radically different from the ones we actually have – a fundamental misunderstanding has occurred and we have not communicated successfully.

Such misunderstandings often happen when patients ascribe negative values to health workers' verbal or non-verbal actions. Consider the traditional 'caring' relation between nurses and patients (Crawford et al. 1998), which I describe in more detail below. Nowadays it is often difficult to satisfy patients' need for attention, care, and communication. Often, it is simply impossible for nurses to stay with patients for a long time, but sometimes patients misunderstand this constraint. Failing to realise that the problem is the system and not the nurse, a patient might misconstrue that the nurse simply does not want to spend much time with him, or is not interested in giving information, displaying empathy, and offering care. Consequently, the patient might think that the nurse does not possess basic attitudes that a 'good' nurse should possess.

The most fundamental link from ethics to communication is that communication is the best tool for solving difficult ethical dilemmas (Davis et al. 1997). The question of how to communicate with patients who do not want necessary medical treatment is very much a question of how one should try to achieve consent that is as well informed as possible (Young 1998). Communication is also necessary in order to determine whether patients' preferences are autonomous, that is, whether they are capable of rational reasoning and sufficiently well informed about their state of health and the consequences of their wishes. Within the practical limits of a given situation, health workers should, therefore, always do their best to communicate relevant information.

Indeed, a good solution to an ethical dilemma will always presuppose good communication. The reason is that a good solution involves agreement, and agreement presupposes a shared understanding of the situation. Here is a typical example from Sanders (2001, 98):

> The paramedic crew has been dispatched to an office building where a 55-year-old woman collapsed at a business meeting. She is alert and oriented, complains of chest pain, and is pale and diaphoretic. The paramedics advise the patient of the possibility of heart attack and the need for immediate care and transport for physician evaluation. She insists on waiting until after the meeting has concluded to seek medical care on her own, and she asks the EMS crew to leave.

Now the initial thing to do in this case is to inform the woman of the danger of not receiving medical treatment and transport. The probability that she will change her preferences is significantly improved if she realises the potential gravity of the health situation. If the paramedics fail to communicate this in the first place, then there can be no communicative way out of the problem. Either the woman will be transported against her will or she will be left on her own. None of these options represents a good solution to the ethical dilemma, but if the paramedics fail to use a communicative strategy, these two options will be regarded as the only possible options.

A second area where communicative challenges arise within the context of an ethical dilemma is situations involving patients or relatives of patients in crises (Nordby 2008c). Health personnel often experience issues of how to communicate with patients who are in shock, despair or intense pain as ethical questions, and they frequently interpret the choice as being one between a close, personal contact and a detached role as a professional health worker, equipped with an 'expert' perspective on the physiological aspects of patients' conditions. What kind of communicative strategy does the person in crisis want? The answer varies from situation to situation, and it is often difficult to understand the preferences of each individual patient or relatives of the patient (Nordby 2008c).

The fact that the choice of 'good' actions often involves communicative strategies and verbal actions should be mentioned as an independent important point. Discussions of ethical dilemmas have traditionally focused on non-verbal actions – body movements that express intentions (Guttenplan 1996). But there is no distinction in principle between reflecting on what is a 'good' non-verbal action and reflecting on what is a 'good' verbal action. In books about patient communication the focus is often on verbal actions; in books about bioethics the focus is traditionally on non-verbal actions. This tendency is in my view unfortunate. I have given some initial examples of how the two areas are essentially linked, and the discussions below can give the reader a more precise understanding of why communication and ethics should not be disconnected.

7. The chapters

Beginning with a wide characterisation of applied philosophy, I have gradually narrowed my focus in order to capture the specific perspective that this book represents. In this last section I shall provide a more detailed presentation of each chapter in order to make it easier for the reader to acquire a holistic understanding of the overall themes of the book.

The aim of 'Meaning and normativity in nurse-patient-interaction' is to discuss communicative challenges that arise in the light of the fact that nurses and patients seldom understand medical concepts in the same way. The fundamental problem can be stated as a problem about concept possession: how is it possible for nurses and patients to share medical concepts despite the diversity of understanding? I use a theory of concepts from cognitive science and philosophy of mind to present a solution to this problem. According to this theory, nurses and patients share the same medical concepts – and thereby understand the same meaning of the language they use – if they are willing to defer to the same normative standards for the application of the concepts. Case studies are used to show that this analysis has striking practical implications for how nurses should improve and secure patient communication.

In 'Interactive and face-to-face communication: a perspective from philosophy of mind and language' I start out by making a general distinction between face-to-face and interactive communication. This, I emphasise, is a distinction that is especially important for health workers working in first-line medical services where interactive communication is used a great deal. I then derive four fundamental communication conditions from recent philosophy of mind and language, and use these conditions to clarify essential similarities and differences between face-to-face and interactive communication. The aim is to give paramedics and other health workers in the first line services a better understanding of these similarities and differences, so that they are in a better position to secure successful communication and avoid misunderstandings.

In 'The analytic-synthetic distinction and conceptual analyses of basic health concepts' I discuss the nature of basic health concepts like *disease, illness and sickness*. Many theorists have attempted to give definitions of these concepts that can function as general standards in patient communication, but as more and more definitions have been rejected as inadequate, pessimism about the possibility of formulating plausible definitions has become increasingly widespread. However, the belief that there can be no plausible definitions since no definitions have received widespread acceptance is an inductive objection and therefore not very conclusive. I argue that an influential argument against the 'analytic-synthetic distinction' from philosophy of language constitutes a more fundamental objection. I use *disease* as an example and show that this argument implies that *disease* and other controversial health concepts do not have analyses grounded in a common language. Stipulative and contextual definitions can have a local significance and play an important role in patient communication, but the normative roles of such definitions are at the same time limited.

'Wittgenstein's theory of conceptual competence and virtue analyses of ethical dilemmas in nursing practice' discusses Ludwig Wittgenstein's philosophy of conceptual competence within the area of nursing ethics. I argue that Wittgenstein's philosophy shares fundamental assumptions with virtue approaches to ethical dilemmas in caring practice, but it is at the same time crucially different. The main difference is that while virtue theories have focused on psychological attitudes like compassion and empathy, Wittgenstein focuses on a person's understanding of concepts like *good* and *wrong*. I discuss how Wittgenstein's position should be understood and show that it has striking implications within health care. According to the analysis I develop, nurses should address ethical dilemmas in patient interaction by focusing on their understanding of ethical concepts in the context of the interaction. Case studies are used to clarify this and other practical implications of Wittgenstein's position.

In 'Truth-telling in doctor-patient interaction' I discuss what it is for doctors to be truth-telling. In the light of Henderson's influential argument that it is impossible to tell patients the whole truth, theorists have recently suggested that the idea of a truth-telling doctor should be connected to a doctor's intention to be sincere. The problem with this kind of intentionalism about truth-telling, I argue, is that truth-telling is a *communicative* concept – a doctor has told a patient the truth only if he has communicated the truth. I discuss how a communicative concept of truth-telling should be understood and use case studies to show that the communicative concept has practical implications that are strikingly different from the implications of pure intentionalism.

In 'The ethical dimension of paramedic-patient interaction' I discuss an ethical dilemma that paramedics and other health workers working in first-line medical services sometimes face. The dilemma can be described as choice between two different action-guiding principles: confronted with a patient who does not wish to receive treatment and transport, should paramedics act in accordance with the patient's preferences or is it correct to force the patient to receive treatment? I show that this dilemma involves a choice between an ethics that focuses on 'good' consequences and a Kantian ethics that focuses on patients' right to decide. I then argue that this dilemma has a practical solution in many emergency cases: if the patient is not autonomous, and if letting the patient decide has serious negative consequences for the patient, then judgements about consequences should overrule the Kantian considerations. This condition, I argue, is met in a range of cases in medical first-line services.

References

Ashcroft R, Lucassen A, Parker M, Verkerk M and Widdershoven G (2005). *Case analysis in clinical ethics.* Cambridge: Cambridge University Press.

Brink D (1989). *Moral realism and the foundations of ethics.* Cambridge: Cambridge University Press.

Chalmers A (2005). *What is this thing called science?* Buckingham: Open University Press.

Crawford P, Brown B and Nolan P (1998). *Communicating care.* Cheltenham: Stanley Thornes.

Dahlberg K, Drew N and Nyström M (2001). *Reflective lifeworld research.* Lund: Studentlitteratur.

Dancy J (1991). *Contemporary epistemology.* Oxford: Blackwell.

Dancy J (2004). *Ethics without principles.* Oxford: Oxford University press.

Davis A, Aroskar M, Liaschenko J and Drought T (1997). *Ethical dilemmas in nursing practice*. Stamford: Appleton and Lange.

Flick U (2002). *An introduction to qualitative research*. London: Sage publications.

Gillon R (2001). 'Telling the truth, confidentiality, consent and respect for autonomy'. In J Harris (ed): *Bioethics*. Oxford: Oxford University Press.

Glaser B and Strauss A (1967). *The discovery of grounded theory: Strategies for qualitative research*. Chicago: Aldine.

Grayling A C (1998). *Philosophy two: Further through the subject*. Oxford: Oxford University Press.

Gubrium J and Holstein J (2002). *Handbook of qualitative interviewing*. Thousand Oaks: Sage publications.

Guttenplan S (1996). *A companion to the philosophy of mind*. Oxford: Blackwell.

Haack S (1995). *Evidence and inquiry: Towards reconstruction in epistemology*. Oxford: Blackwell.

Habermas J (1984). *The theory of communicative action*. Boston: Beacon Press.

Henderson L (1935). 'Physician and patient as a social system'. *New England journal of medicine*, 35, 21–35.

Higgs R (2006). 'On telling patients the truth'. In H Kuhse and P Singer (eds): *Bioethics: An anthology*. Oxford: Blackwell.

Hollis, M (1994). *The philosophy of social science*. Cambridge: Cambridge University Press.

Kuhn T (1970). *The structure of scientific revolutions*. Chicago: University of Chicago Press.

Kuhse H and Singer P (2001). *A companion to bioethics*. Oxford: Blackwell.

Kushner T and Thomasma D (2001). *Dilemmas for medical students and doctors in training*. Cambridge: Cambridge University Press.

Nordby H (2008a). 'Lay conceptions of disease and illness in doctor-patient interaction'. *Theoretical medicine and bioethics*, 6, 357–370.

Nordby H (2008b). 'Values, cultural identity and communication'. *Journal of intercultural communication*, 2, 30–47.

Nordby H and Nøhr Ø (2008c). 'Communication and empathy in an emergency setting involving persons in crisis'. *Journal of trauma, resuscitation and emergency medicine*, 5, 25–31.

Nordby H (2009). 'Scepticism and internalism'. *Canadian journal of philosophy*, 1, 35–54.

Nordenfelt L (2001). *Health, science and ordinary language*. Amsterdam/New York: Rodopi.

Peacocke C (1992). *A study of concepts*. Cambridge/MA: MIT Press.

Raz J (2005. *The practice of value*. Oxford: Oxford University Press.

Sanders M (2001). *Mosby's paramedic textbook*. St Louis: Mosby

Sperber D and Wilson D (1991). 'Loose talk'. In S. Davis (ed): *Pragmatics: A reader*. Oxford: Oxford University Press.

Silverman J, Kurtz S and Draper J (2004). *Skills for communicating with patients*. Oxford: Radcliffe publishers.

Wittgenstein L (1969). *On certainty*. Oxford: Blackwell.

Wulff H (1992). 'Does the philosophy of medicine exist?' *Theoretical medicine*, 13, 67–77.

Young R (1998). 'Informed consent and patient autonomy'. In H Kuhse and P Singer (eds): *A companion to bioethics*. Oxford: Blackwell.

Yamada S, Slingsby B, Inada M and Derauf D (2008). 'Evidence-based public health: a critical perspective'. *Journal of public health*, 16, 169–172.

Chapter 2

Meaning and normativity in nurse-patient-interaction

Summary It is a fundamental assumption in nursing theory that it is important for nurses to understand how patients think about themselves and the contexts they are in. According to modern theories of hermeneutics, a nurse and a patient must share the same concepts in order to communicate beliefs with the same content. But nurses and patients seldom understand medical concepts in exactly the same way, so how can this communicative aim be achieved in interaction involving medical concepts? I use a theory of concepts from recent cognitive science and philosophy of mind to argue that nurses and patients can share medical concepts despite the diversity of understanding. According to this theory, two persons who understand medical language in different ways will nevertheless possess the same medical concepts if they agree about the normative standards for the applications of the concepts. This entails that nurses and patients normally share medical concepts even though patients' conceptions of disease and illness are formed in idiosyncratic ways by their social and cultural contexts. Several practical implications of this argument are discussed and linked to case studies. One especially important point is that nurses should seek to make patients feel comfortable with deferring to a medical understanding. In many cases an adequate understanding of patients presupposes that nurses manage to do this. Another implication is that deference-willingness to normative meaning is not equivalent to the actual application of concepts.

Deference-willingness should rather be thought of as a precommunicative attitude that it is possible for patients who are not fully able to communicate to possess. What is important is that nurses and patients have the intention of conforming to the same meaning.

1. Introduction

It is a fundamental assumption in modern nursing theory that nurses and other health personnel involved in caring practice should be able to understand how patients think of themselves and the contexts they are in (Orlando 1961; Travelbee 1971; Parsons 1979; Enelow et al. 1996). It is obviously sometimes difficult or even impossible for patients to communicate, and sometimes the quality of care does not depend on an essential understanding of what beliefs, thoughts and feelings patients have. However, the fact that there are cases of this kind is consistent with the idea that there are very many cases of nurse-patient-interaction in which it is important for nurses to understand and communicate with patients (Lewis 1978; Crawford et al. 1998; Nordby 2004).

From a nurse's perspective, understanding a patient can be conceived of as a comprehensive process that gradually reveals more of the nature of the patient's condition of disease or illness and his/her beliefs about this condition. Obviously, this does not mean that successful nurse-patient-interaction always depends on a very detailed, complete understanding. The idea of a complete understanding should rather be thought of as an abstract ideal that it is possible to approximate to a greater or lesser degree, depending on the context of interaction (Warnke 1987).

The distinction between the process of understanding and the aim of understanding is essential in modern hermeneutics, and is primarily associated with the philosopher Hans-Georg Gadamer (1975; 1994). According to Gadamer, the ideal aim of understanding is achieved when two persons adopt the same cognitive perspective – the same beliefs, thoughts and opinions – because they both find it rationally compelling. The understanding that is formed and gradually changes in the process of achieving this aim is not based on agreement, but on a partial recognition and internalisation of another person's set of beliefs (Gadamer 1975; Bleicher 1980).

The first aim of this chapter is to show that there is a tension between this hermeneutic conception of understanding and the different ways patients conceive of medical concepts. It has been extensively documented that patients understand concepts related to disease and illness in different ways (Lupton 1994; Nettleton 1995). While health professionals normally have a competent medical understanding, patients typically have a vague or partial understanding, shaped by their idiosyncratic social and cultural contexts. Furthermore, a professional understanding is formed holistically by medical theory, which most patients have limited knowledge of (Radley 1964). It might therefore seem that the hermeneutic aim of understanding can seldom be achieved in nurse-patient-interaction involving medical concepts: since nurses and patients normally understand such concepts in different ways, it is difficult to understand how they are able to communicate beliefs involving the same concepts.

The second and principal aim of the chapter is to use a theory of concept possession to argue that nurses and patients can share medical concepts even when they do not understand the concepts in the same way. According to this theory, which has become influential within recent philosophy of mind and cognitive science, persons with a competent understanding of a concept have explicit knowledge of what the concept applies to. Consumers of a concept – persons with a partial understanding – will nevertheless possess the same concept as those who have explicit knowledge, if they are willing to defer to the correct understanding of the concept (Putnam 1975; 1981; Peacocke 1992).

I will emphasise that this analysis applied to the area of nursing practice is consistent with the reasonable idea that it should not be necessary for nurses and patients to have an identical understanding in order to be able to communicate beliefs when communication is important. It is sufficient that they are, on the basis of verbal or non-verbal language, willing to defer to the same meaning of the concepts that are employed in the interaction.

Several practical implications of this argument are discussed on the basis of case studies. An especially important one is that nurses, when they are entitled to think that their understanding represents the normative meaning, should seek to create a context in which patients feel comfortable about deferring to this understanding. By displaying attitudes like empathy and compassion nurses can make patients feel that they are recognised and respected as persons with a disease or illness. This, in turn, can make patients more wiling to adopt nurses' understanding of medical language.

A second implication is that nurses and patients can share medical concepts in cases where patients have partially lost their ability to communicate; it is possible for patients to meet the conditions for being consumers even though they cannot fully manifest their understanding. A third implication is that deference-willingness is not a behavioural capacity. It should rather, in a sense to be explained, be thought of as a precommunicative attitude: patients need to have the attitude in order to be able to possess and communicate medical concepts.

2. Shared beliefs as an aim of understanding

Knowing how to communicate is to have implicit or explicit knowledge of conditions that must be met in order for communication to happen. Many of these conditions will differ depending on the area of discourse, but some remain important across different contexts. This section clarifies the general idea that understanding in human interaction in a fundamental sense involves shared beliefs involving the same concepts. In the next sections I will apply this idea in a discussion of nurse-patient-communication.

The general study of understanding is often labelled hermeneutics. Hermeneutical concepts apply within areas where the object of study has two kinds of properties. Firstly, the object in question needs to have content. The aim of the process of understanding is to achieve knowledge of what this content is. Secondly, the object needs to have perceptually accessible properties that express its content. It is on the basis of interpretation of these expressions that an interpreter forms beliefs about the essential content of the object.

Objects of hermeneutic studies include works of art and literature, but within the social sciences the central objects of focus have been human beings. A hermeneutical approach to persons aims to understand the motives, thoughts and feelings that underlie observable human actions. Such actions can be verbal speech-acts but also other forms of body language. What is important is that the actions are intentional, that they express subjective states like beliefs and feelings. It has been common to think of a person's total set of such subjective states as his overall horizon, as the total perspective he has of himself and the world around him (Warnke 1987; Mueller-Vollmer 1986).

A central assumption in classical hermeneutics has been that two persons' horizons are never identical, and that it is important for an interpreter not to let interpretation be colored by the interpreter's subjective horizon. According to classical hermeneutics, when trying to understand another person it is therefore important to disregard one's own horizon. The aim of the interpretative process is to form a neutral, objective understanding that is independent of one's own perspective (Critchley and Schroeder 1998; Mueller-Vollmer 1986).

In the last decades of the 20th century an alternative theory of hermeneutics, primarily associated with the writings of Hans-Georg Gadamer (1975; 1986; 1994), has challenged the classical ideal of understanding. Like earlier theorists, Gadamer accepts that our cognitive and emotional perspectives constitute our subjective horizons holistically. But Gadamer does not accept that this implies that the aim of understanding is to achieve an objective understanding that is independent of the interpreter's horizon. The problem with this view, Gadamer holds, is that it is impossible to form such an understanding: 'We are always within the situation', always within 'the range of vision that includes everything that can be seen from a particular vantage point' (Gadamer 1986, 269). Trying to achieve an objective, neutral understanding is like trying to get a view from nowhere (Nagel 1986).

All understanding must be based on interpretation, and all interpretation must be made on the basis of the particular horizon an interpreter has (Gadamer 1975; 1986).

According to Gadamer, the fact that interpretation cannot be based entirely on intersubjectively accessible facts and general, objective knowledge means that interpretation is essentially contextual, that it is always connected to a particular context:

> [The aim of understanding] is to understand the phenomenon itself in its unique and historical concreteness. Even if general experience is involved, the aim is not to confirm and expand these general experiences (Gadamer 1975, 6).

Consequently, Gadamer holds that the process of understanding is an interaction between an interpreter's horizon and the person he/she tries to understand. As this process goes on two persons who gradually understand each other adjust their horizons to new aspects of the horizons that are uncovered. Fundamental understanding is in this sense 'always the fusion of horizons' (Gadamer 1986, 272), always a comprehensive overlap of shared beliefs and thoughts (Gadamer 1975; 1986; Nagel 1986; Critchley and Schroeder 1998).

It should be emphasised that this view is not equivalent to the idea that an interpreter actually forms another person's beliefs. A person's beliefs are in an obvious sense only his/her beliefs, reported by using indexical expressions like 'I' in reports like 'I believe that ...' Obviously, if a patient reports 'I am in pain', then this will not cause a nurse to form a belief the nurse expresses by' I am in pain'. What the patient and the nurse share is the content of the belief, the content that *the patient is in pain*. Accordingly, I will from now on understand the idea of shared beliefs in the following way: two persons X and Y share a belief about Y if they both believe of Y that p, where the proposition p describes the content of the belief in question.

Gadamer's rejection of the idea that there exists an objective basis for interpretation and his alternative analysis of understanding have become influential within applied philosophy in the last decades. In particular, the conception of the process of understanding as a gradual fusion of horizons has been used as an analytical framework for discussing theoretical challenges related to communication and understanding in many different areas (Bleicher 1980; Davidson 1984; Smith 1997; Green 2000). In the following I will focus on challenges related to the use of medical concepts in nursing practice.

3. Patient conceptions of disease and illness

In this section I argue that there is an apparent incompatibility between the hermeneutic aim of understanding and the different ways patients conceive of illness and disease.

Patients' understanding of medical concepts related to disease and illness has been analysed in two ways. Firstly, theorists have made conceptual analyses of basic concepts like *disease*, *illness* and *sickness* in order to elucidate how the contexts patients and health personnel are in determine how the concepts are understood. In particular, attention has been paid to the fact that patients are typically medical laypeople, that they do not have detailed knowledge of the application conditions of medical concepts. Patients' understanding is instead shaped by their idiosyncratic social and cultural contexts. Holistic concepts like *medical anthropology*, *holistic health* and *social role theory* have often been used to explain how this happens (Mechanic 1968; Lupton 1994; Nettleton 1995; Nordby 2004a).

Secondly, theorists have taken an empirical approach to the diversity of understanding. Extensive studies have shown that patients and medical professionals typically understand basic medical concepts in different ways and explained the ways in which they do so. Nettleton provides an extensive discussion of empirical research and concludes that

> [...] understandings and beliefs about health clearly vary among different groups. This variation is largely accounted for by the

social, cultural, biographical and economic context within which individuals are located (Nettleton 1995, 66).

There is an apparent conflict between this diversity of understanding of medical concepts and the hermeneutical framework of understanding that was presented above. The problem can be formulated as follows: it is often important that a nurse understands what beliefs a patient has about himself and the situation s/he is in. According to the hermeneutical framework, understanding what beliefs a patient has is a matter of sharing beliefs with the patient. Furthermore, when two persons share beliefs, then these beliefs involve the same concepts. For instance, if a nurse and a patient both believe that sciatica can cause pain, then their beliefs involve the same concepts *sciatica, can, cause* and *pain*. But patients often do not have a very good medical understanding of a concept like *sciatica*. So how can the hermeneutic aim of understanding be achieved in interaction involving this and other medical concepts?

The problem can also be stated in connection with language. If a patient means *sciatica* by the word 'sciatica' then s/he and the nurse expresses the same concept by the word. If a patient does not mean *sciatica* then s/he expresses an alternative concept. In that case the patient and the nurse do not express the same beliefs by sentences involving the word 'sciatica', and they will not be able to understand how the other thinks about sciatica and conditions related to this state.

The scope of the problem of understanding should not be restricted to interaction involving verbal language. It is possible for the problem to arise whenever a patient's behaviour represents subjective intentional states, and where the content of these states involves concepts. In such cases the patient's behaviour expresses the idiosyncratic meaning of his concepts, and when this meaning involves medical concepts that are formed by the patient's special context, it is difficult to understand how it is possible for the patient as a layperson to communicate these concepts to a nurse. The problem of understanding is a general problem that arises whenever patients' intentional behaviour, regardless of whether or not it is verbal, expresses medical concepts that are understood in idiosyncratic ways. For the sake of simplicity, I will in the following focus on verbal language, but it will be clear how the arguments generalise to other forms of communication.

The problem of securing communication of concepts has not received much attention in discussions of understanding in nursing practice. The reason seems to be as follows: it is a truism that a nurse has an adequate understanding of a patient when s/he has an adequate conception of what the patient's perspective is. But it is generally assumed that this can only be a conception that approximates the patient's perspective, since it is impossible to adopt the patient's perspective completely (Lewis 1978; Parsons 1979; Crawford et al. 1996; Enelow et al. 1998).

It is true that it is impossible to grasp a patient's understanding in the sense that it is impossible to understand the patient's overall use of language. This total use is formed holistically by the patient's past and present context, which is inaccessible to a nurse. But what is special about the hermeneutical conception is that it makes a sharp distinction between two notions of understanding: a patient's understanding of language s/he uses can be thought of as his/her overall use of the language, but also as the concepts s/he expresses. The fundamental assumptions connected to the latter notion are that patients express beliefs by means of language, and that the content of these beliefs is made up of concepts (Guttenplan 1996; Becthel and Graham 1998). The condition of identity of concepts follows directly from these assumptions. In order for a nurse and a patient to understand each other, they have to be able to share beliefs involving the same concepts; a degree of similarity is insufficient.

More could be said about the philosophical nature of this problem of understanding, but this would fall outside the focus of this paper. I will, however, argue that the hermeneutical framework and the facts about the diversity of understanding are compatible despite appearances to the contrary. I will argue that they can be combined if one accepts that patients are, in a sense to be explained, consumers of medical concepts.

4. Degrees of conceptual competence

The idea that there can be degrees of conceptual competence and its implications for the status of laymen conceptions are often associated with the writings of Hilary Putnam (1975; 1981; 1996). Putnam was originally concerned about defending the idea that speakers with limited knowledge of natural kind concepts mean the same as experts when they use natural kind terms. His most famous example involves a person who is ignorant of the chemical nature of water. Such a person will nevertheless, according to Putnam, mean *water* by 'water'.

According to Putnam, this case falls under a general description of 'division of linguistic labour' (1975, 14). Putnam (1975, 13) claims that every linguistic community

> [...] possesses at least some terms whose associated 'criteria' are known only to a subset of speakers who acquire the terms, and whose use by the other speakers depends upon a structured cooperation between them and the speakers in the relevant subsets.

Putnam's fundamental idea is that even though some speakers do not qualify as competent speakers, they mean the same as those with a competent understanding if they are willing to defer to the correct use. The correct understanding provides a normative standard, and when a person defers to the correct use he shows that he intends to use the word in accordance with this standard. The person is, in short, a consumer of the conceptual competence that the expert has (Putnam 1975). On the other hand, if a person is not willing to defer to what he thinks is the correct use, then s/he should be conceived of as someone who does not wish to use the word in accordance with the normative meaning. Such a person has decided to understand the word in an idiosyncratic way that is not necessarily consistent with the standard use.

I will further clarify implications of the theory of conceptual competence below, but it should already be clear that it suggests a straightforward solution to the problem of securing nurse-patient communication of medical concepts. For according to the theory, even though a nurse and a patient understand medical language differently, they express the same concepts if the patient is willing to defer to the correct medical explanations of what the language means. For instance, a deference-willing patient and a nurse will associate the same concept *diabetes* with the word 'diabetes', even though the patient does not have detailed knowledge of what diabetes is. More generally, the beliefs nurses and patients express by whole sentences involving the word 'diabetes' involve identical concepts if they are willing to defer to the same standard meaning of the words that the sentences involve.

A further example will help to clarify the argument:

> A patient has been hospitalised after having suffered a severe stroke. Medical personnel tell him various things about his condition. One sentence that is used is 'Your blood pressure is now much more stable'. The patient has no more than a vague understanding of what blood pressure is, but the doctor is busy and the patient is tired, so the patient does not ask for more information about the meaning of the term. Later a nurse attends to the patient. The patient asks the nurse what the term 'blood pressure' really means, and the nurse provides a more detailed explanation. This explanation becomes part of the patient's overall conception of what blood pressure is. The concept he expresses by 'blood pressure' is therefore identical to the nurse's standard medical concept.

Nurses involved in caring practice will for various reasons often provide explanations of the nature of states related to patients' disease or illness. In such cases, if the patient accepts the explanations, as patients undoubtedly very often do, then it follows from the theory of conceptual competence that the nurse and the patient share the same concepts.

The theory has comprehensive implications for how one should think of understanding and communication in nursing practice.

As emphasised above, the problem of understanding does not merely arise in interaction involving verbal language. The theory of conceptual competence applies in a similar way to cases where a person expresses concepts in non-verbal ways. Applied to nurse-patient-interaction the general implication of the theory is that patients show that they possess medical concepts if they show that they are willing to defer to relevant medical explanations. The hermeneutic condition of understanding is met no matter *how* patients display deference-willingness to normative meaning.

The fact that concepts can be expressed in a variety of ways has a further implication that is important in nursing practice. Nurses often encounter patients who do not have the ability to communicate fully. The underlying cause can be an injury or state of disease or illness, but also a physical disability of a more or less permanent nature. In such cases patients are typically unable to explicate their overall understanding of beliefs they wish to communicate. It is important to note that if nurses needed comprehensive knowledge of how patients understand their beliefs in order for communication to succeed, then it would be impossible for these patients to communicate their beliefs successfully. But nurses do not need such comprehensive knowledge according to the theory of conceptual competence. It is sufficient that the minimal condition of deference-willingness is met, and in number of cases patients who are unable to fully explicate their understanding will be able to show that they accept explanations provided by the nurse.

Some patients are obviously not able to communicate at all, and in these cases communication cannot be used to achieve understanding. It is therefore a further issue how well a patient must be able to communicate in order for understanding to be facilitated by communication. This 'how-well' question is a general question that has to be addressed in different ways depending on the theoretical and methodological framework that is used, and it would fall outside the argumentative focus of this paper to pursue the question.

However, I think it is important to note that, according to the theory of conceptual competence, a key aspect of the 'how-well' question concerns deference to medical explanations: if a patient is able to show that he accepts a nurse's explanation of a medical term, then he also associates the standard concept with the term. According to the theory of conceptual competence, this threshold condition for concept possession should have an important role in discussions of communication in nurse-patient-interaction.

It has often been held that a solution to a theoretical problem is essentially incomplete unless it provides, implicitly or explicitly, an explanation of why the problem was felt to be a problem in the first place (Wittgenstein 1953). In the present context an important part of this explanation is that we do not have a clear pretheoretical grasp of the distinction between two ways of conceiving of a patient's understanding of medical language. As noted above, nurses and patients very seldom use medical language in exactly the same way. But they can still understand medical language in the same way in the sense that they associate the same concepts with the same terms. It is this latter concept of understanding that the present argument is focused on.

The main aim here is not to present conclusive arguments in favour of the theory of conceptual competence. What I have wanted to show is that the problem of fundamental understanding can be solved on the basis of the theory. An important consequence is that if someone claims that it is overwhelmingly difficult to secure shared beliefs in nursing practice, then an explanation of why the theory should be rejected has to be provided. Developing such an explanation is a challenging task, especially in the light of the fact that a large number of theorists have thought that there are convincing arguments in favour of the theory (Putnam 1981; Peacocke 1992; Guttenplan 1996; Pessin and Goldberg 1996; Nordby 2004b).

It should also be mentioned that there is an obvious sense in which the theory of conceptual competence is supported by common sense. Ehen we encounter laypeople who use medical terms, we do not ordinarily hesitate to ascribe to them beliefs involving standard medical concepts. If someone who does not have detailed medical knowledge of what hypertension is says 'My mother's hypertension is getting worse', we do not normally hesitate to ascribe to the person the belief that his mother's hypertension is getting worse, involving the concept *hypertension*. Furthermore, the theory is supported by the strong intuition we have that patients should not have to learn detailed medical theory in order to be able to communicate with health professionals they encounter. It seems too demanding to claim that communication requires that the medical concepts employed in the interaction are understood in exactly the same way.

If one wants to show that the theory of conceptual competence is not supported by common sense, it is necessary to show that the theory has counter-intuitive implications that outweigh the appeal of the idea that patients should not need expert knowledge of medical concepts in order to be able to share concepts with health personnel. But it is difficult to understand how there could be a convincing objection of this kind. As long as the theory is grounded in our ordinary practices of ascribing concepts to laypeople, then any counterintuitive consequence must be implicit in these practices. It must be possible to discover, simply by reflecting on the practices, that they have consequences that are unacceptable. But it is, at least *prima facie*, natural to think that they do not. It is more reasonable to believe that the implications of what we ordinarily find acceptable will be conceived of as reasonable as well (Burge 1986; Pessin and Goldberg 1996).

This point is particularly important in connection with the aspect of the producer-consumer distinction that concerns deference-willingness to normative meaning. I have shown that the distinction implies that we should make a sharp distinction between patients who are willing to conform to medical explanations and patients who are not. Only patients in the first category should be thought of as consumers of the correct understanding. Some might object that this has the following unreasonable consequence: consider two patients, A and B, who have a similar, incomplete understanding of a medical expression. When A is confronted with a nurse who provides a more detailed explanation of this expression, he defers to this explanation. When B is presented with a similar explanation, he is not willing to defer. In such a case the producer-consumer distinction implies that A and B do not associate the same concept with this expression, not only after the encounters with the nurses, but also before. However, at this earlier stage A and B had the same beliefs about the term; we could even imagine that A and B are similar in very many other respects. So is it not unreasonable to maintain that they associate different concepts with the expression?

The problem with this objection is that it fails to acknowledge the strong appeal of the idea that deference-willingness is part of our understanding of the concepts we possess. As long as A is willing to defer, then there is a relevant difference between A and B in the sense that A has a substantial psychological attitude that B does not have. In Peacocke's words, we should distinguish deference-willingness to normative meaning 'from the quite different case of an individual's taking over a word from his community and using it in his own individual sense' (Peacocke 1992, 29). Patient A fundamentally conceives of himself as a member of our linguistic community, in which the expert understanding constitutes a common norm. B, on the other hand, has chosen to understand the expression in a special, non-standard way. There is therefore a deep, relevant difference between patients A and B.

In fact, the suggestion that A and B possess the same concept has to be weighed not only against this difference, but also but against our overall practices of ascribing beliefs. Granted that B does not possess the standard concept since he manifestly makes it clear that he has chosen to understand the expression in his own non-standard way, the suggestion that A and B possess the same concept implies that A possesses B's alternative concept. But as long as we normally do not hesitate to ascribe medical concepts to patients who do not have a complete understanding, then this implies that we should revise these practices; it would always be incorrect to ascribe standard concepts to patients who are willing to defer, as very many patients are undoubtedly willing to do.

It is also important to bear in mind the problems one confronts if one tries to determine non-standard concepts in alternative ascriptions. If patients possess special concepts that correspond to their idiosyncratic, incomplete understanding, comprehensive knowledge of their understanding would be required in order to correctly ascribe the individual concepts they possess. But such knowledge would be overwhelmingly difficult to achieve in most cases of nurse-patient-interaction. We therefore need to ask: is it plausible to believe that the implications of the idea of deference-willingness, an idea that in it self has a strong appeal, should lead us to revise our ordinary practices and instead ascribe non-standard concepts? I have not meant to argue conclusively that the answer is no, but it is difficult to understand how there could be a convincing argument for an affirmative answer to this question.

There are, in sum, good reasons for holding that the theory of conceptual competence should be used to analyse understanding and communication in caring practice. Consequently, it is justified to believe that nurses and patients often share medical concepts when the interaction involves such concepts.

5. Applications

In this final section I discuss some further practical implications of the argument I have presented. One of them concerns what nurses should do in order to secure understanding. Consider the following case:

> A nurse attends to an elderly patient who needs regular care. During an encounter the patient complains about feeling warm and feverish. The nurse observes that the temperature in the patient's bedroom is rather high and suspects that this is the cause, but in order to be on the safe side she takes his body temperature. She informs the patient that 'Your temperature is slightly above normal, but it is very likely that this is due to the warm room so I do not think that you have a fever'. The patient does not

understand this and says to himself: 'She does not think that I have fever, but I must surely have since my body temperature is above normal'.

In this case the patient does not defer to the nurse's use of the term 'fever'. The belief that the patient expresses by the word 'fever' therefore involves an alternative concept of fever that matches the patient's special understanding. If the nurse had chosen a more empathetic course of action, then there is a good chance that the patient would have adopted the nurse's understanding. The nurse could have said something like this: 'Your temperature is above normal, and I fully understand that you are feeling feverish. However, in medicine it is common to restrict the term 'fever' to temperatures above normal that are caused by internal bodily states and not an increase in temperature in the external environment.'

Expressing such an emphatic attitude would also have helped to avoid possible misunderstandings in the future. One might imagine that the patient as described in the case later calls some relatives and says 'The nurse denied that I have a fever but I know that I have.' As a consequence the relatives become worried about the patient's condition and the quality of the care he receives.

More generally, if a nurse is entitled to think that s/he has a correct understanding, and if there are no special reasons why a patient should not adopt this understanding, then the nurse should seek to create a context in which the patient is comfortable about deferring to the understanding. It is reasonable to assume that a friendly and empathetic attitude often is the crucial factor for establishing a common platform of shared concepts that can be used as a basis for communicating beliefs and thoughts.

I emphasised above that the significance of deference-willingness to normative meaning should not be restricted to cases in which patients are able to fully communicate. It can sometimes be difficult for patients to express their overall understanding of their condition of disease or illness, and it can be difficult for a nurse to determine whether s/he has succeeded in communicating information that is considered to be important. The theory of conceptual competence implies that a nurse can sometimes avoid these difficulties: by being explicit about explanations of medical language a nurse can make reasonable inferences about the nature of patients' beliefs. If a patient is able to show that he accepts an explanation of a medical concept, then the nurse is entitled to think that the patient possesses this medical concept. On the other hand, if it is not reasonably clear that a patient accepts the correct explanation, then the nurse is not justified in concluding that the patient possesses the concept. It is unnecessary for nurses to obtain detailed knowledge of patients' overall understanding in order to make plausible judgments about the content of their beliefs.

Another important implication of the theory of conceptual competence is that deference-willingness to normative meaning is a preconceptual and precommunicative attitude:

> A person is hospitalised after having sustained a head injury. When she awakens she has a headache and is nauseous. A nurse explains to the patient that she has suffered from a brain concussion and asks how she is feeling. The patient says that she has a headache, but informs the nurse that 'There must be something else wrong with me as well, for I am feeling very nauseous'. The nurse explains to the patient that a brain concussion can often cause nausea. As a consequence the patient widens her understanding of her concept *brain concussion*.

In this case the patient thinks of the nurse as someone who knows more about the concept of brain concussion that she does herself. The patient does not have conceptual knowledge of the full content of her own concept *brain concussion*, and her attitude of being willing to defer to the correct understanding is therefore preconceptual. Furthermore, the attitude is precommunicative in the sense that the patient needs to have the attitude in order to be able to communicate with the nurse. The fact that the patient accepts the further explanation about nausea means that her thoughts involved the concept *brain concussion* even before the nurse provided the explanation. At this stage the patient did not know that brain concussions can cause nausea, but her willingness to accept medical explanations entailed that she nevertheless possessed the concept. If the patient did not have this attitude, then she would not have understood that the nurse expressed the belief that a brain concussion can often cause nausea, involving the concept *brain concussion*.

The fact that that deference-willingness to normative meaning is precommunicative has a further implication: when it is difficult for patients to express their beliefs they might still, in their own minds, assent to medical explanations of their states of disease or illness provided by a nurse. In such cases patients defer, and thereby possess the same concepts as the nurse, even though this attitude has not been expressed in behaviour. The important consequence of this is that nurses should not think of the condition for shared concept as a condition of *observable* assent to implicit or explicit explanations of what medical concepts mean. A patient who has not shown that he accepts an explanation of a medical concept should not necessarily be understood as a person who possesses an alternative concept.

At the same time it is not always the case that a patient who is able to present his idiosyncratic understanding chooses to do so. A patient might think of a nurse as rigid medical authority and as a consequence prefer to not present and defend a non-standard conception of what a medical concept means. It is reasonable to assume that this sometimes happens in interaction involving basic health concepts like *disease*, *illness* and *sickness* that do not have precise medical definitions (Worhall and Worhall 2003). Patient conceptions of these concepts are often significantly different from conceptions used by health professionals (Lupton 1994; Nettleton 1995). In particular, the fact that the concepts have a traditional usage outside the medical profession implies, as extensive empirical research has confirmed, that patients commonly think that they are entitled to have their own 'non-professional' understanding (Mechanic 1968; Helman 1984). In interaction involving everyday medical concepts nurses should therefore be aware of the possibility that patients may not present their alternative conceptions. In such cases, patients' use of terms like 'disease' and 'illness' express, contrary to what seems to be the case, non-standard concepts that correspond to their alternative understanding.

A third implication of the theory of conceptual competence is that shared beliefs do not constitute a guarantee against misunderstandings. But such misunderstandings occur because a nurse and a patient understand one and the same concept in different ways, not because they have different concepts. What is important is that the nurse and the patient are willing to accept the same meaning when the differences emerge. It is therefore possible for misunderstandings to occur as long as the differences remain undetected, i.e. as long as the nurse and the patient do not think that they misunderstand each other. An example can illustrate the point:

> A mother takes her child to a health centre because of blisters. She is told that the child has chickenpox, and that the best thing to do is to have the child rest. Some time later the mother calls the health centre and informs a nurse that the child is getting worse, and she says that 'I think it was a mistake to not give her antibiotics'. The nurse explains to the mother that chickenpox is caused by a virus, and that antibiotics will not help. The mother adjusts her understanding of the concept of chickenpox in accordance with the nurse's explanation.

In this case the mother does not merely believe that her child has chickenpox after she has been corrected. The fact that she accepts the nurse's explanations means that her beliefs involved the concept *chickenpox* even before she was corrected; she genuinely believed that her child had chickenpox, and she genuinely believed that antibiotics cure chickenpox. If the nurse had been aware of the latter belief then she would have explained to the mother that this belief was false, but the nurse did not know that the mother had the mistaken belief.

This point about the possibility of misunderstanding should also be mentioned as a separate point in connection with the general plausibility of the arguments I have presented. If the arguments had implied that there is no way misunderstandings can occur then that would be problematic, since that would not correspond to how we ordinarily conceive of nurse-patient-communication. It should be possible for nurses and patients to misunderstand each other, even when they are members of the same linguistic community. This is precisely what the present arguments imply; a nurse and a patient who speak the same language in the sense that they express the same concepts by the same expressions can nevertheless understand these concepts in different ways. It is therefore incorrect to claim that the arguments does not allow for misunderstanding.

A further discussion of this and other aspects of the arguments would fall outside the scope here. My aim has been to show that the availability of the theory of conceptual competence means that the sceptical view that nurses and patients are unable to share medical concepts is unjustified. I have also indicated how the theory implies that understanding can be secured in different forms of nurse-patient-interaction. It is reasonable to assume that it is nurses involved in daily caring practice who have the best capacity for applying and refining these implications further.

References

Bechtel W and Graham G (1998). *A companion to cognitive science*. Oxford: Blackwell publishers.

Bleicher J (1980). *Contemporary hermeneutics: Hermeneutics as method, philosophy and critique*. London: Routledge.

Burge T (1986). 'Intellectual Norms and Foundations of Mind'. *Journal of Philosophy*, 83, 697–720.

Crawford P, Brown B and Nolan P (1998). *Communicating care: The language of nursing*. Cheltenham, UK: Stanley Thorne Publishers.

Critchley S and Schroeder W (1998). *A companion to continental philosophy*. Oxford: Blackwell publishers.

Davidson D (1984). *Inquires into truth and interpretation*. Oxford: Clarendon Press.

Enelow A., Forde D. and Brummel-Smith K (1996). *Interviewing and patient care*. Oxford: Oxford University Press.

Gadamer H G (1975). *Truth and method*. New York: Seabury Press.

Gadamer H G (1986). 'The historicity of understanding'. In K. Mueller-Vollmer (ed): *The hermeneutics reader: Texts of the German tradition from the enlightenment to the present*. Oxford: Blackwell publishers.

Gadamer H G (1994). *Literature and philosophy in dialogue*. Albany NY: State University of New York Press.

Garland K L (1978). *Nurse-patient communication*. Foundations of nursing series. Iowa: Dubuque.

Green G (2000). *Theology, hermeneutics, and imagination: The crisis of interpretation at the end of modernity*. Cambridge: Cambridge University Press.

Guttenplan S (1996). *A companion to philosophy of mind*. Oxford: Blackwell publishers.

Helman C (1984). *Culture, health and illness*. Oxford: Butterworth-Heinemann.

Lupton D (1994). *Medicine as culture*. London: SAGE Publications.

Mechanic D (1968). *Medical sociology*. New York/London: The Free Press.

Nagel T (1986). *The view from nowhere*. Oxford: Oxford University Press.

Mueller-Vollmer K (1986). *The Hermeneutics reader: Texts of the German tradition from the enlightenment to the present*. Oxford: Blackwell publishers.

Nettleton S (1995). *The sociology of health and illness*. Cambridge: Polity Press.

Nordby H (2004a). 'The importance of knowing how to talk about illness without applying the concept of illness'. *Nursing philosophy*, 5, 30–40.

Nordby H (2004b). 'Concept Possession and Incorrect Understanding'. *Philosophical explorations*, 7, 55–72.

Orlando I. J (1961). *The dynamic nurse-patient relationship*. New York: National league for nursing.

Parsons V and Stanford N (1979). *Interpersonal interactions in nursing*. Menlo Park: Addison-Wesley.

Peacocke C (1992). *A study of concepts.* Cambridge, MA: MIT Press.

Peplau H E (1952). *Interpersonal relations in nursing practice.* Toronto: Putnam's sons.

Pessin A and Goldberg S (1996). *The twin earth chronicles.* New York/London: M.E. Sharpe.

Putnam H (1975). *Philosophical papers.* Cambridge: Cambridge University Press.

Putnam H (1981). *Reason, truth and history.* Cambridge: Cambridge University Press.

Putnam P (1996). 'The meaning of 'meaning''. In: A. Pessin and S. Goldberg (eds): *The twin earth chronicles.* New York/London: M.E. Sharpe.

Radley A (1994). *Making sense of illness.* London: Sage publications.

Smith N (1997). *Strong hermeneutics: Contingency and moral identity.* London: Routledge.

Travelbee J (1971). *Interpersonal aspects of nursing.* Philadelphia: Davis.

Warnke G (1987). *Gadamer: hermeneutics, tradition, and reason.* Stanford: Stanford University Press.

Wittgenstein L (1953). *Philosophical investigations.* Oxford: Blackwell publishers.

Worhall J and Worhall J (2003). 'Defining disease: Much ado about nothing?' *Analecta husserliana,* 72, 33–55.

Chapter 3

Interactive and face-to-face communication: a perspective from philosophy of mind and language

Summary The aim of this chapter is to derive fundamental communication conditions from central assumptions in recent philosophy of mind and language, and then use these conditions to clarify essential similarities and differences between face-to-face and interactive communication. The analyses are to a large extent made on the basis of participant observations and dialogues with students in a further education course for medical paramedics, but the conclusions should be of interest to anyone who has a pedagogical interest in understanding the nature of the two forms of communication. The arguments set out have both a descriptive and a normative dimension. They are descriptive in the sense that they aim to give a philosophical analysis of successful communication; they are normative in the sense that they seek to understand how communication can be improved. The chapter concludes that the philosophical analysis presented constitutes a plausible conceptual framework for analyzing empirical phenomena related to face-to-face and interactive communication.

1. Introduction

Lecturers, supervisors and other persons with teaching responsibilities in modern education programs are often involved in two forms of communication: face-to-face communication, in which the participants in a communicative process can observe each other and the wider context of communication, and interactive communication, in which communication happens through some interactive communication channel. Dialogues with students in traditional, physical classrooms are typical examples of the first kind of communication; supervision and discussions via internet-based programs like 'Classfronter' are typical examples of the second.

It is obvious that both face-to-face and interactive communication can involve fundamental challenges for communicators, but it is not so clear exactly how these challenges should be understood and related to each other. An important theoretical question is therefore this: to what extent are the communicative challenges involved in the two forms of communication similar, and to what extent are they essentially different?

A thorough analysis of all the potentially relevant aspects of this question would require a very comprehensive discussion. The obvious reason is that the question can be discussed from different perspectives, and that it is unreasonable, at least *prima facie*, to give one of these perspectives conceptual or epistemic priority (Davies 1998; Peacocke 1998). A better suggestion is that the similarities and differences between face-to-face communication and interactive communication can be elucidated in different ways, and that a variety of analyses can jointly contribute to a better, overall understanding of the nature of the two forms of communication.

My primary motivation for exploring the nature of face-to-face and interactive communication has been the need to understand communicative challenges that confront students in a national further education program for medical paramedics. As the person responsible for one of the courses in this program I have, from a pedagogical and theoretical point of view, attempted to analyze the various forms of interaction paramedics are involved in. I have, in particular, sought to address two questions: what are some of the fundamental problems of understanding paramedics confront when they encounter patients and other health personnel in face-to-face situations? How are these problems similar to, but also different from, the challenges they confront when they communicate interactively via radio or telephone with other health personnel such as nurses in acute medical communication centers?

The aim of this chapter is to address some important aspects of these questions on the basis of recent philosophical theories of speech acts and concept possession (Guttenplan 1996; Bechtel and Graham 1998). Within the theoretical framework I develop, I make a fundamental distinction between four communication conditions: firstly, speaker and audience (in a wide sense) need to share a common language that can be used to convey and understand a belief. Secondly, the audience must realize that the speaker has the intention of communicating this belief. Thirdly, speaker and audience must not associate beliefs and thoughts that are literally expressed in language with very different sets of other beliefs and thoughts. And finally, the experiences, motives and values that an audience ascribes to a speaker must not be radically different from the experiences, motives and values that a speaker intends to express.

I will argue that this philosophical framework is completely general but also particularistic. That is, the four conditions can be used to show how face-to-face and interactive communication involve some of the same fundamental communicative processes, but the conditions can also be used to illuminate crucial differences. This fact, I will argue, constitutes a plausible argument for using the conditions as a conceptual framework for analyzing empirical phenomena related to the two forms of communication. Moreover, the fact that the framework is suitable for understanding and explaining the two forms of communication constitutes an independent justification for the framework itself, as a genuine theory of communication.

In the last part of the chapter, I examine the question of how it is possible to avoid various forms of misunderstanding that occur when one or several of the four communication conditions are not met. This discussion is to a large extent based on ideas that have been central within modern philosophical hermeneutics (Bleicher 1980; Mueller-Vollmer 1986; Smith 1997). I focus particularly on Gadamer's (1975) idea of the aim of understanding as a 'fusion of horizons' and argue that in order to avoid poor communication, it is imperative that speakers are aware of various intrinsic aspects of the cognitive and emotional perspectives audiences have. I conclude that this and other implications of the arguments I present should be of interest to anyone who wants to acquire a more philosophical understanding of the nature of face-to-face and interactive communication.

2. Background

'Nasjonal Paramedic Utdanning' (http://paramedic.hil.no/) is a national further education course for health personnel working as paramedics in the national health services in Norway. The program consists of six courses, four of which focus mainly on issues directly related to medicine, one on legal issues and one on communication and ethics.

The need for focusing on communication in the program is obvious. In their daily work as paramedics the students are to a large extent involved in interpersonal relations where empathy, understanding and dialogue are important factors for securing successful interaction. With respect to the especially important relation between paramedics and patients, it is crucial that paramedics are able to understand adequately how patients experience and think about their states of disease, illness or sickness. Their choice of verbal and non-verbal behavior must be based on justified beliefs about the emotional and cognitive perspectives patients have on their condition of disease or illness (Enelow, Forde and Brummel-Smith 1996; Nordby 2004a; Nordby 2006).

A detailed analysis of the diversity of communicative contexts paramedics face in interaction with patients and other health personnel falls outside the scope of this chapter. The important point I will focus on is that paramedics are involved in two forms of communication that are essentially different from each other. Firstly, they are involved in many direct, face-to-face encounters with patients, relatives of patients and other health personnel – situations in which they are able to observe not only the persons they communicate with but also the wider context of communication. When communicators are able to observe each other in this way, the obvious consequence is that it is possible to use more than uttered words as interpretative clues. Interpretation can also be made on the basis of non-verbal behavior and other observable aspects of the communicative context (Nordby 2004b). The significance of this consequence is obvious. Normally, when we seek to understand other persons we rely on literal interpretation. As Burge (1979, 88) observes, 'literal interpretation is *ceteris paribus* preferred' in ordinary discourse. For instance, if a speaker says 'It is raining', audiences normally assume that the speaker, as long as he means to be sincere, expresses the belief that it is raining involving the concepts *it, is* and *raining* that are literally expressed by the words he utters.

The qualification 'normally' is important. Sometimes certain aspects of a situation constitute good reason for being sceptical about literal interpretation, as in the case of incongruent communication involving a definite mismatch between verbal and non-verbal behavior. By being sensitive to the potential importance of non-verbal interpretative clues, communicators can avoid incongruent communication and other forms of poor communication that can occur when there is a mismatch between what is strictly speaking *said* and what is more generally displayed (Eide and Eide 2004). In such cases of experienced inconsistency, attentive audiences use the wider context to form special non-literal and complex interpretations that do not correspond directly to the words that a speaker utters (Davidson 1984). Furthermore, it is a widespread view that there are no observable aspects of face-to-face communicative contexts that are irrelevant in principle for determining the non-literal meaning of verbal speech acts (Bezuidenhout 1997; Cappelen and Lepore 2005). Face-to-face interpretation is essentially holistic; interpreters' beliefs about the meaning of speakers' utterances are based on assumptions about of all sorts of contextual observations and all sorts of assumptions about speakers' social and cultural contexts.

Face-to-face communication has received most attention in the health care literature focusing on interaction between health personnel and patients, but interactive communication – here defined as communication that does not involve a face-to-face encounter – is often equally important for paramedics (Tjora 1997). When an ambulance is called out, it has received an interactive appeal from an Acute Medical Communication center (AMC-center) where emergency nurses who cooperate with ambulance coordinators have answered an emergency call ('113' in Norway). This interactive appeal has several elements, including a precise a description as possible of where the patient is, a categorization of the acuteness of the assignment according to a code, and an indication of the nature of the patient's state of injury, illness or disease.[1]

Furthermore, while patients are being transported there is often extensive interactive dialogue between paramedics and the AMC-center. The paramedics often provide information about the patient's state of illness or disease, they sometimes ask for medical supervision, and they sometimes require further back-up assistance from other medical units. There are, in fact, a wide range of aspects related to patients' conditions that are of potential significance in this interactive communication. From the perspectives of all the parties involved, the experienced success of the paramedic-patient interaction will often depend heavily on adequate interactive communication.

It should already now be emphasized that when I distinguish between face-to-face communication and interactive communication in this way, I do not mean to argue that the two types of communication involve communicative processes that are different in principle. On the contrary, I believe that the assumptions I make are consistent with

---

[1] An important motivation for providing information about the patient's condition is that the paramedics can prepare themselves mentally and in practical terms for the situation that awaits them.

the plausible view that communication is a contextual, interpretative process, and that the difference between face-to-face and interactive communication fundamentally is a difference of degree. The reason this is an important point to make is that some might infer from the above that I rely on unjustified assumptions about some underlying principled distinction, but this is not the case. All I am presupposing is that we have a reasonable clear idea of what the differences between face-to-face and interactive communication are.

More could be said about face-to-face and interactive communication and the particular ways in which paramedics are involved in these forms of communication, but this would fall outside the limits here. For the present argumentative purposes, it is sufficient to clarify the basic nature of two forms of communication. I assume, in particular, that I have made it clear that face-to-face communication and interactive communication must involve some different communicative challenges. In the following, I will first develop fundamental communication conditions that are relevant for understanding communication in general, and then use these conditions to shed light on relevant differences.

3. A philosophical perspective

In trying to understand some of the fundamental communicative challenges that paramedics confront in their daily work as health personnel, it has been important to make extensive observation studies in ambulances and AMC-centers. These studies have given me valuable knowledge of how the students in the further education course experience and try to solve problems of communication. At the same time it is important to remember that although observations of human behavior and interaction must necessarily provide the basis for deciding whether communication succeeds or fails in a given context, such observations alone cannot establish whether communication succeeds. Conclusions about the status of a communicative process must always be made on the basis of assumptions about the nature of communication. Traditionally, these assumptions have focused on how the 'external' – behavior and context – must match the 'inner' – the subjective and private (Davidson 1984; Bezuidenhout 1997; Cappelen and Lepore 2005). The traditional idea has been that a speaker has successfully communicated an 'inner' mental state S to an audience if, and only if, the audience understands that the speaker intends to use verbal or non-verbal actions to convey state S to him.

Of course, making such communicative assumptions is something we do more or less unconsciously all the time in ordinary discourse, and even if the aim is nothing more than to explicate our common everyday assumptions, we have in effect started to clarify a theory of communication. Indeed, the difference between common sense theories of communication and the philosophical perspective I will apply here is not meant to be one of principle. The aim is rather to locate assumptions that (a) appeal to our ordinary ideas and (b) can be used to understand the fundamental challenges that face-to-face and interactive communication involve.

The theoretical framework I will use in seeking to achieve this twofold aim is grounded in a modern tradition within cognitive science and philosophy of mind and language (Guttenplan 1996; Bechtel and Graham 1998). According to theories that fall within this tradition, verbal and non-verbal actions are conceived of as intentional language acts that express beliefs and thoughts. Beliefs and thoughts are in turn thought of as psychological attitudes to propositions involving mental concepts (Burge 1979; Peacocke 1992). For instance, the sentence 'Water quenches thirst' is normally used to express the belief that water quenches thirst involving the three concepts *water*, *quenches* and *thirst*. When a speaker associates these concepts with the sentence, communication of the concepts has succeeded if, and only if, the audience understands that the speaker intends to communicate a belief involving these concepts.

It should be emphasized that this does not mean that an audience must necessarily think that is it correct to understand a language act in the same way as a speaker. For communicative purposes, all that is required is that the belief that an audience thinks that a speaker intends to communicate really is the belief the speaker intends to communicate. Questions about the objective and normative status of the meaning of language acts are therefore not directly relevant for questions of communication; whether communication happens must be determined on the basis of considerations of how speaker and audience understand each other, not on the basis of considerations of how it is correct to understand a given language (Nordby 2006).[2]

This point is of particular importance in discourse involving disputed concepts with unclear application conditions, like the basic health concepts *disease, illness* and *sickness* (Mechanic 1968; Nettleton 1995; Worhall and Worhall 2003). Health professionals sometimes encounter patients who do not understand these concepts in ways that correspond to influential conceptions within the health services, but if a paramedic tries to adopt a patient's understanding for communicative purposes, exchange of concepts can happen even if the patient's understanding is regarded as controversial or even incorrect.

A second and more philosophical point that should be made about the framework of communication that I will use, is that I do not mean to argue that it constitutes the only possible way of analyzing communication. Basically, what I am relying on is that the framework represents a fundamental and influential way of understanding human interaction. I presuppose, in particular, that the assumption that successful communication involves successful exchange of subjective states has an intuitive, immediate appeal that is grounded in our ordinary communicative practices. Of course, in everyday communication it is not common to think of exchange of thoughts and other subjective states as communicative processes, but the reason why the assumption is plausible is not that it aims to capture a process that we are consciously aware of in ordinary discourse. The reason is rather that as long as we conceive of communication as a rational activity, then we have to think of understanding and communication

---

[2] It is in general a sound methodological principle that issues of understanding and communication are not subject to questions about normativity in the way questions of truth and knowledge are.

in cognitive terms: our understanding of the language we use, and the way we try to communicate our concepts to others, cannot be reduced to observable behaviour. As McDowell notes,

> [...] to learn the meaning of a word is to acquire an understanding that obliges us subsequently – if we have occasion to deploy the concept in question – to judge and speak in certain determinate ways, on pain of failure to obey the dictates of the meaning we have grasped' (McDowell 1994, 160).

McDowell's claim is illuminating, not only because it is reasonable in itself, but also because McDowell ascribes it to the later Wittgenstein. In contrast to the tradition that McDowell's interpretation of Wittgenstein is framed within, Wittgenstein is sometimes described as a modified behaviorist. According to this behaviorist interpretation, communication is essentially an observable activity within 'language-games', an activity that can be fully explained by referring to how we conform to language rules in different contexts (Kripke 1982).

Whether or not it is (contrary to what McDowell thinks) correct to ascribe some kind of behaviorist 'third person' perspective to Wittgenstein, is an important question of exegesis, but it would fall outside the scope here to address it. For the present purposes it is more important to think of behaviorism as a genuine source of challenge to cognitive analyses of communication. Independently of what Wittgenstein writes, some might argue that all versions of behaviorism are not obviously false, and that I have not showed why the cognitive framework of communication I have adopted here is more plausible than all these versions.

Is important to say something briefly about this objection, first and foremost because the choice of framework has substantial different practical consequences. Consider as an example a patient who utters the sentence 'I am in pain' and a paramedic who comes to assistance. A behaviorist will typically think of this as a complete communicative process and claim that further explanations that refer to 'underlying' subjective states and audiences' mental interpretations of these states are irrelevant, superfluous or 'quasi' explanations that fall outside the realm of proper psychological explanations.

There are in my opinion two main problems with this view. Firstly, and as indicated above, if McDowell is correct, then it is possible to think that the way we understand words and communicate meaning is derived from our use of language, and at the same time think that explanations of underlying mental phenomena are important. According to McDowell, what Wittgenstein is opposed to is not mental explanations *per se*, but a certain way of conceiving of the relation between 'private' subjective states and observable actions. It is only if one starts out with a classical Cartesian first-person perspective that one is easily led to think that this dualism involves overwhelmingly difficult epistemic and metaphysical obstacles (Burge 1979; Nordby 2004c). The problem with behaviorism as a response to the Cartesian tradition is that the position inherits the same dualistic way of thinking. The only difference is that behaviorism starts from the other end – from the 'outside' – and then claims that it is only this perspective that we have 'real' epistemic access to. Behaviorism is a general doctrine that is grounded in a positivistic idea of what counts as elements in scientific explanations of communication.

Secondly, objections to the scientific status of cognitive analyses of communication often seem to rest on the idea that there is only one 'proper' level of psychological explanation. However, there is no good reason for holding that this is so. It is true that it is possible, on one level, to explain communication from a third-person perspective. And from this perspective it is correct to say that communication has succeeded if an audience manifests appropriate behavior as a response to actions performed by a speaker. But accepting that this is correct is compatible with holding that there is more to say about underlying mental processes from other perspectives.

Consider again the above example of a patient who utters 'I am in pain' and a paramedic who comes to assistance. How are we to understand this as a communicative process? We find it overwhelmingly natural to assume that the patient really is in pain (as long as he is sincere), that his utterance expresses his experience of being in pain, and that he intends the paramedic to understand that he is in pain (as long as his utterance is not merely an expression of pain) and so on. It is equally natural to assume that the reason the paramedic comes to assistance is that he thinks that the patient is in pain. This idea about the patient's state of illness is derived from the fact that the patient used the sentence he used, and probably other interpretative clues like signs of pain. In short, the paramedic forms a belief about the patient's state of mind on the basis of observable properties of the context. Again, this does not depend on a special Cartesian picture of the mental, or on the idea that interpretation is a conscious process. It is simply a natural way of widening a more narrow third-person explanation of what communication involves.

Hopefully, this defense of the plausibility of the cognitive framework has indicated why it has a strong appeal, and why proponents of other approaches therefore face formidable challenges. Obviously, much more could be said about communication as a fundamental philosophical concept, but that would fall outside the aim here as long as my main focus is the application of the framework within health care. In the next section I will argue that theories of speech acts and concept possession can potentially shed theoretically interesting light on face-to-face and interactive communication, and that they can be used to analyze crucial differences within a completely general framework. I have explained how the framework focuses in a comprehensive way on verbal and non-verbal speech acts, but I have also indicated how it implies that an observable context can play a crucial role in interpretation. In the following I will first focus on the issue of general significance and then discuss the idea of an observable context in more detail.

4. Communication conditions

Clarifying how communication can succeed or fail is equivalent to clarifying communication conditions – conditions that must be met in order for successful communication to happen. In order to understand communicative challenges within the framework I have outlined, I will make a fundamental distinction between four conditions. The first is that communication requires a common language:

(i) In order for an audience to understand a speaker, it is necessary that they share a platform of shared concepts.

Here I use the expression 'speaker' in a wide sense to mean someone who has a belief, thought or other concept-involving psychological attitude that he wishes to communicate to an audience (one or several persons). Since audiences are unable to grasp speakers' thoughts and beliefs directly, these subjective states have to be expressed in language acts that can be seen, heard or observed and interpreted in other ways. As emphasized above, this can be all sorts of intentional behavior, but for the sake of clarity I will in the following primarily focus on verbal speech acts. Thus, in order for an audience to be able to understand that a speaker expresses a given belief, it is necessary that the speaker and the audience understand the sentence that the speaker uses in a sufficiently similar way, so that they associate the same concepts with the words that the speaker uses (Cappelen and Lepore 2005).

The qualification 'sufficiently similar' is important. When I claim that speaker and audience must have a common language, I do not mean that they have to understand this language in the same way in the sense that they use it in exactly the same 'language games' (Wittgenstein 1953). It is sufficient that their understanding is so similar that that they associate the words that are used with the same concepts (Burge 1979; Peacocke 1992; Guttenplan 1996).

This, in effect, presupposes that the conditions for the sharing of concepts are weaker than the conditions for sameness of understanding. It is obvious that communicators must have some similar understanding of a word in order to associate the same concept with it – the understanding that the audience has must to some extent approximate the speaker's understanding.[3] But this leaves open what a sufficiently similar understanding is, and exactly what the threshold condition for shared concepts is has been a disputed issue (for a discussion of this, see Nordby 2004c).

I will not presuppose any specific view on this issue here, but I will rely on the widespread idea that it is unnecessary that communicators use a word in exactly the same way in order to associate the same concept with it. The main reason why this idea is reasonable is this: we very seldom use language in exactly the same ways; there are normally differences due to our respective social and cultural contexts. So if we needed an identical understanding in order to share concepts, we would, in fact, seldom be able to exchange beliefs and thoughts involving the same concepts. Furthermore, laypersons should not need complete expert competence regarding the application conditions of a term in order to express the same concept as persons who have expert competence (Putnam 1981; Pessin and Goldberg 1996). If that were the case, laypersons within a given area of discourse would be unable to communicate with experts (consider again the area of health care and the relation between patients and medical doctors). This is a counterintuitive consequence, and it constitutes a good reason for being sceptical about the view that a platform of shared concepts requires an identical understanding.

The second communication condition I wish to focus on is more straightforward:

(ii) In order for a speaker to be able to communicate a belief, he needs to have the attention of the audience.

The idea is as follows: a speaker might express a belief, used a language that the speaker and the audience have a sufficiently similar understanding of and think it has reached the consciousness of the

---

[3] As emphasized above, this can be an understanding that the audience thinks is correct in general but also an understanding that is employed for communicative purposes. The important point is that the understanding that the audience employs must approximate the speaker's understanding.

audience. It can nevertheless happen that the audience fails to realize that the speaker intends to communicate this belief. The reason for this may be lack of attention, problems of interpretation due to a chaotic situation, or an impaired capacity for rational reasoning (a patient might be in a state of shock or under the influence of drugs). But the problem may also be of a more technological nature, e.g. computers that do not work so that audiences are unable to use them as interactive communication tools.

It is important to bear in mind that in order for a misunderstanding of this kind to occur, the speaker must be unaware of the communicative problems. The speaker must genuinely believe that he has the attention of the audience, that there is no significant communicative 'noise' or disruption; otherwise he would not be sincerely attempting to communicate a belief. An example can be used to illustrate the point:

> Paramedics encounter a patient who has taken a large amount of paracetamol. Relatives have called 113, and the patient himself, in a confused and agitated state, makes it clear that he does not want to be taken to hospital. In order to persuade the patient that treatment in hospital is necessary, the paramedics try to inform the patient about the physiological effects of paracetamol and they tell him that large doses of paracetamol can lead to serious irreversible damage to the liver. They hope that this information will lead the patient to change his mind, but this does not happen. Consequently, the paramedics decide that there is little use in trying to persuade the patient, and they begin to consider more complicated strategies for securing necessary transport and treatment.

In this situation it was evident that the paramedics assumed that the information about the negative health effects of large doses of paracetamol had reached the consciousness of the patient. However, it soon became evident that this had not happened. When the patient calmed down and his relatives told him what the paramedics had said, the patient realized the gravity of the situation and made it clear that he wanted to go to the hospital after all. In the first place, because of his confused state and the stressful encounter with the paramedics, the patient did not form the belief that the paramedics intended to communicate and thought that it was important to communicate.

If we manage to avoid the two forms of misunderstands that occur when conditions (i) or (ii) are not met, does this mean that communication has succeeded? Not necessarily. Even if speaker and audience have a platform of shared concepts, and even if the speaker has the attention of the audience so that the message that he intends to communicate actually reaches the consciousness of the audience, it might still happen that the audience associates this message with beliefs and thoughts that are very different from the set of beliefs and thoughts that the speaker associates with the message. This third form of misunderstanding corresponds to a third communication condition:

> (iii) The wider set of beliefs and thoughts that an audience as-
> sociates with a belief that is directly expressed in language must
> not be radically different from the wider set of beliefs and thoughts
> that the speaker associates with this belief.

As Davidson (1987, 449) notes, interpretation always 'rests on vague assumptions about what is and what is not shared' by speaker and audience, and problems typically arise when assumptions about what is shared beliefs turn out to be incorrect. Of course, if communicators' perspectives are so radically different that they influence the semantic interpretation of the language that a speaker uses, then the misunderstanding that arises is a misunderstanding of the first kind (i). In such cases speaker and audience do not even have a common language. A misunderstanding of the third kind requires that the message that is literally expressed by language is understood, that the communicators have a sufficiently similar understanding of the words that are used in the sense explained above. The problem that can still arise is that the beliefs that surround this message are radically different. An example can illustrate the point:

An AMC-nurse tells a patient who has called 113 that 'The ambulance is on its way'. The patient forms the belief that the ambulance is on its way, but he then forms a further belief – the belief that the ambulance will arrive very soon within the next few minutes. The patient expresses disappointment when the ambulance arrives after 30 minutes.

In this case communication of the belief that the ambulance is on its way has succeeded. The AMC-nurse has the attention of the patient, and they both associate the concepts *the, ambulance, is, on, its* and *way* with the sentence 'The ambulance is on its way'. The problem is that communication has failed in the wider sense that the AMC-nurse does not associate the belief that the ambulance is on its way with the belief that the ambulance will arrive within a few minutes.[4] The patient, however, forms this association. He grasps the content of the message that the nurse expresses literally in words, but he then forms further associations that are radically different from the way the nurse intends this message to be understood.

The qualification 'radically different' is important here. Two persons never associate the beliefs and thoughts they form with other beliefs and thoughts in exactly the same way; there will always be some different associations as long as interpretation is shaped by social and cultural context (Burge 1979; Davidson 1984; Smith 1997). The important point is that there are many cases in which the associations that are formed are so different that poor communication occurs. From the perspectives of speakers, it is the beliefs that it is most important to communicate that are ordinarily expressed literally in words; that is why communication of these beliefs is normally straightforward. It is when speaker and audience understand what is not strictly speaking *said* in significantly different ways, that a misunderstanding of the third kind (iii) occurs.

---

[4] When the condition of a patient is perceived as not being acute the ambulance is not required to adopt 'code one' which is the code for acute situations, and it might take some time before it arrives (but outside central areas it might take some time even if the code is 'code one').

Is communication ensured if we manage to avoid the three forms of misunderstanding that correspond to communication conditions (i)–(iii)? We might think so, but this is because we sometimes tend to forget that communication is not always a rational activity. In addition to beliefs and thoughts that are true or false, there are many other subjective states that are important in human interaction. The fourth and final communication condition is meant to capture the fact that we sometimes communicate psychological states that are essentially different from beliefs and thought that are true or false:

(iv) The values, emotions and other non-conceptual subjective states that an audience ascribes to a speaker must not be different from the values, emotions and other non-conceptual states that the speaker intends to communicate.

By 'values, emotions and other non-conceptual subjective states' I mean states that cannot be ascribed as beliefs or thoughts that involve concepts. When we think about communication we often tend to focus on such states, on attitudes we ascribe by saying things like 'S believes that p' or 'S thinks that p' where 'p' is a concept-involving proposition. For instance, when I say 'S believes that snow is white', I ascribe to S the attitude of believing in a proposition involving the three concepts *snow, is* and *white* (which is true if snow is white and otherwise false). It is easy to forget that we sometimes intend to communicate psychological states that are not attitudes to propositions. Personal values are not attitudes to propositions, it makes no grammatical sense to say 'S values that p' and replace for 'p' propositions that are true or false depending on how the world is. Personal values are rather attitudes to 'forms of living' (Wittgenstein 1953; Johnston 1989), to the ways we wish to live our lives and the activities we like to participate in (Dancy 1996).

The same applies to emotions and other personal experiences. The way I feel a certain pain, or the way I have a visual impression of a computer in front of me, cannot be directly experienced by another person. I can attempt to report and communicate my experience by using a sentence that I think is true or false ('I am in pain', 'I have the impression of seeing a computer in front of me'), but this sentence is not identical to the state I talk about and have privileged first-person access to. The state is a pure subjective experience, not a belief or thought about something (Rosenthal 1991).

Understood in this way, the significance of (iv) becomes similar to that of (iii). We often try to communicate our personal values and experiences to other persons, but sometimes our audiences ascribe to us states that are different from those we intend to communicate. For instance, a patient who uses emotional vocabulary like 'I am in pain' will normally be interpreted as expressing a state with a certain qualitative 'pain' content. If this interpretation is wrong – if the pain that the paramedic thinks that the patient feels is very different from the qualitative nature of the pain the patient feels – then a misunderstanding of the fourth kind has occurred.

Values that are attitudes to forms of life or activities are subject to the same problems of interpretation. In discourse between persons from different social or cultural contexts the values that are ascribed may be different from the values that the communicators have. It is reasonable to assume that this sometimes occurs in paramedic-patient interaction. A patient who is perceived as a person who appreciates that the paramedics are acting in a certain way might in fact be a patient who endorses an alternative course of action. Typical cases include interaction between elderly people and younger paramedics who have a more 'modern' way of life. In one case observed by the author of this book, a paramedic consequently addressed an elderly patient by his first name, even though it was fairly evident that the patient would have appreciated an alternative course of action (e.g. he introduced himself using his surname).

This last communication condition (iv) might seem to inflate the philosophical framework of speech acts and concepts, but this is not the case. On the contrary, since the first three conditions focus entirely on concept-involving beliefs and thoughts, it is possible to formulate a fourth condition that captures the remaining 'subjective' and qualitative dimension of human communication. The philosophical framework I have outlined leaves room for this further condition precisely because it makes a sharp distinction between concept-involving and non-concept-involving subjective states.

5. Implications: interactive and face-to-face communication

I am not going to argue that the four conditions I have presented represent the only possible way of analyzing communication. Holding that they are reasonable is consistent with holding that there are other conditions that are important as well. In fact, I do not even mean to provide a direct argument for the view that the conditions offer a plausible analysis of how poor communication can occur. What I primarily wish to focus on is their explanatory power, particularly the way they can be used to shed light on the similarities and differences between face-to-face and interactive communication.

If we start with the first condition (i), i.e. having a common language, how is this condition relevant for understanding the nature of the two forms of communication? The basic distinction to be made in connection with (i) is that between what a word means and what a speaker means. An utterance heard on the phone or a sentence read on a computer screen means something – it has a semantic content. But when an audience is confronted with a speaker the immediate question for the audience is as follows: what is the mental state – belief, thought or value – that the speaker has and intends to communicate?

This difference of focus corresponds to two different ways of conceiving of a speech act. The activity that is performed interactively is a pure language act; the social context of the act is not part of the meaning of the act. From the perspective of an audience, the aim is to understand the proposition expressed by the language shared by the speaker and the audience. The focus must be explicitly or implicitly on meaning, and the relevant interpretative activities correspond to the scope of philosophy of language – to philosophical questions about the meaning of language.

Face-to-face communication, on the other hand, is a social activity that essentially belongs within pragmatics and philosophy of mind. The question that confronts face-to-face communicators is this: what is the belief that the speaker in this context uses language to express? This is not a semantic question about the meaning of the words *per se*, but a question about the psychological nature of the relevant mental states of the speaker.

Even though the interpretative activities involved in the two forms of communication in this way correspond to different philosophical disciplines, it is important to recognize that the activities are similar in the sense that they both involve literal interpretation. That is, we normally assume that words that are used literally express the concepts communicated. We assume, for instance, that the word 'dog' in interactive communication means *dog*, just as we assume that a speaker who uses the word 'dog' expresses a belief involving the concept *dog*. In this sense there is an important similarity between face-to-face and interactive communication, and the requirement that communicators need to have a common language can be used to understand challenges related to concept communication within both forms of communication.

At the same time it is important to bear in mind that there are sometimes good reasons for not accepting literal interpretations, and in such cases the differences between face-to-face and interaction communication become more significant. In order to show why this is so it is important to distinguish three kinds of expressions. The first is what might be considered words with vague or unclear application conditions. Many words that are used in everyday discourse do not have precise definitions, and the meaning explanations speakers give often differ even though they are members of the same linguistic community (Burge 1979; 1986).[5] Three of the most disputed words in the area of health care are 'disease', 'illness' and 'sickness' (Lupton 1994; Radley 1994; Worhall and Worhall 2001), but the point is of course general. There are countless vague or abstract words that communicators tend to understand in significantly different ways.

The fact that we commonly use vague words has an important consequence: different conceptions of what words mean are normally easier to detect face-to-face than interactively. There are at least three reasons why this is the case. Firstly, face-to-face communication more often than interactive communication involves substantial dialogue over time in which communicators realize that they do not have a similar understanding. Furthermore, when differences emerge and receive attention, audiences who are interested in communicating tend to adjust their conceptions of what speakers mean.

Secondly, it is sometimes evident from the body language or verbal behavior of a person that he does not share the understanding of another person. If a doctor tells a patient who is feeling ill that it has not been establish that he has a disease, and if the patient thinks that the doctor has a very narrow, rigid understanding of 'disease', the patient's body language may manifest incongruent communication: even though the patient *says* that he accepts the doctor's opinion, the patient's body language or other aspects of the communicative context indicate that he disagree.

Thirdly, in face-to-face communication speakers have time, and it is often natural, to explicate in some detail how they understand words they conceive of as controversial. In particular, speakers often

---

[5] A meaning explanation is here understood as the explanation a speaker would give if he was asked to explain what a word applies to. Meaning explanations are very seldom conceived of as complete descriptions of what a word means; we do not consider them as sentences that capture the whole meaning of the term we are asked to explain. They are rather statements that capture central aspects of a word's meaning. Compare, for instance, the explanation 'The word "dog" applies to a group of mammals with four legs' with the explanation 'The word "dog" applies to an animal my grandmother has'. Only the first statement is normally conceived of as a meaning explanation.

provide direct or indirect meaning explanations of words they think the audience has an incomplete understanding of.

Again, these points must be understood as *prima facie* principles that do not cover all cases. For instance, speakers regularly provide meaning explanations in interactive communication, consider an explanation of what an 'essay' is that a teacher distributes to his students via the internet. And face-to-face communication does not always involve extensive rational dialogue and proper explanations of theoretical or technical terms that are conceived to be important, as the above 'paracetamol case' clearly illustrates. However, it is surely the rule and not the exception that it is easier to detect and influence different conceptions of what a word means in face-to-face communication than in interactive communication.

This also applies to a second kind of words that can be termed 'qualitative words'. Qualitative words are words that refer to private, individual experiences, or subjective states that have a significant personal element. Typical examples are words that denote states like pain, nausea or dizziness, but the category, as I understand it here, also includes emotional vocabulary like 'love', 'compassion' and 'empathy' that are used to communicate states that do not so clearly refer to determinate conscious experiences. The important point is that these words also have a subjective, private dimension that it can be difficult to detect in communication.

Communicative challenges related to the use of qualitative words are to a large extent similar to the challenges related to unclear words, but qualitative words have an additional dimension: an audience has by definition only indirect access to a speaker's first-person experiences, but it is these experiences that constitute the reference and thereby the individual meaning of qualitative words. Qualitative words report these experiences, but they can only function as interpretative clues to the underlying nature of the experiences. This does not necessarily mean that the experiences are completely hidden from an audience; there are few modern traditions in philosophy of mind that hold that emotional states are fully independent from behavior (Rosenthal 1991; Davies 1995; Guttenplan 1996).

The important point is that there must be *some* independence; there are not many theorists today who accept the extreme and classical behaviorist doctrine that experiences are identical to behavior (Ryle 1949). And if we accept the modern, more modest view that experiences are partly displayed in behavior, then it is reasonable to assume that communication of qualitative words more often succeeds in face-to face communication than in interactive communication. Normally, facial expressions or other forms of observable body language constitute part of the content of the experiences that a speaker intends to communicate.

The third category of words that deserve attention is technical or theoretical words. In face-to-face encounters it is sometimes sufficient to watch a person's eyes in order to discern whether theoretical vocabulary represents meaningless sounds or not. Furthermore, in face-to-face interaction it is possible to use various forms of body language as specialized communicative tools. A good example is the non-verbal dialogue in AMC centers between nurses and ambulance coordinators. While talking to patients on the phone, they are able to observe each other and use body language – language that patients do not observe – as part of the basis for deciding what to do. An ambulance coordinator might for instance hold up two fingers to suggest to the nurse that the ambulance should be called out under 'code 2'. If the nurse nods while the patient is on the line, the ambulance coordinator normally proceeds to call up an ambulance under 'code 2'.

There is also a further aspect of the communication of technical words that is essentially different from the communication of unclear words and experiences. The fact that technical words have a standard, normative meaning means that it is possible to make a principled distinction between experts who have a complete, correct understanding and laypeople who have an incomplete understanding. Within recent philosophy of mind, it has been a widespread view that if a layperson is willing to defer to an expert's correct understanding of a word, then he possesses the same concept as the expert even though he does not have a complete understanding. Burge expresses this view in an illuminating way when he writes that

> [...] wherever the subject has attained a certain competence in large relevant parts of his language and has assumed a certain general commitment or responsibility to the communal conventions governing the language's symbols, the expressions the subject uses take on a certain inertia in determining attributions of mental content to him (Burge 1979, 114).

It is only when a person with an incomplete understanding is unwilling to defer to the normative meaning of a word that he should be understood as someone who has chosen to associate the word with his own individual concept that does not correspond to the correct, normative understanding. Deference-willingness is in this sense a precommunicative attitude: laypeople need to have this attitude in the first place in order to be able to possess the same concepts as experts who possess and fully understand the correct, standard concept.

The fact that this point is valid only when the expert-layperson distinction applies has an important implication: from the perspective of a speaker who has a competent understanding, it is often easier to secure a platform of shared concepts by using words with precise application conditions than by using unclear, everyday words that do not have standard, normative definitions. The reason is that audiences normally think they are entitled to understand the latter words in special, idiosyncratic ways if there is no profession that knows what the correct understanding is (Helman 1984; Lupton 1994).

More generally, communicators tend to think that they are justified in understanding and using unclear or vague expressions in accordance with how they have learned them in their particular social and cultural contexts, even though they know that other speakers sometimes use them in other ways in other contexts. In such cases the idea of deference-willingness does not apply: communicators from different contexts will stand face to face and be unwilling to revise their understanding.[6] But when one of the parties is perceived as being an expert on the application of a word within a given area – e.g. the way students often think of their teachers – the non-expert will normally defer and thereby possess the same concept as the expert.

If one seeks to apply this theory of deference-willingness, the strategy will obviously work only if it is possible to give the audience a sufficient understanding and if the audience is really willing to defer. The latter condition is particularly important. Even if there are standard application conditions for a term, this does not help if the audience thinks of the speaker as a strict authority and consequently does not defer to his explanations. From the perspective of a speaker with a competent understanding who faces an audience who does not have a complete understanding, it is therefore necessary to create a situation where the audience feels comfortable deferring to the normative meaning in order to secure a platform of shared concepts. Furthermore, it is reasonable to assume that this aim is easier to achieve face-to-face than interactively. Often a simple smile, a friendly gesture or other form of body language is sufficient for creating an atmosphere in which audiences think of speakers not only as experts, but as *sympathetic* experts. In this deep philosophical sense, it is easier to secure communication of concepts in face-to-face relations than in interactive relations.

6. Further implications

So far I have focused on implications of the first communication condition (i), but as emphasized above, meeting (i) can only be a

---

[6] Consider again a doctor who tells a patient that he has not been able to locate any underlying disease. The patient, we might suppose, thinks that he must have a disease, and thinks that the doctor has a very narrow understanding of 'disease'. An important part of the reason why such an attitude is widespread is that the patient thinks that he is entitled to use 'disease' in the way he has learned the word in his special social and cultural context. This point generalizes to countless words with non-standard application conditions.

necessary condition for meeting the three further conditions (ii)–(iv). When I claim that two persons must understand a language in the same way, what I mean is that they must understand it in the same way in general. Obviously, when a speaker does not have the attention of an audience, speaker and audience do not understand the language *act* that is performed in the same way there and then. What the second communication condition (ii) was meant to capture is the idea that in order for the communication of a belief to succeed, the attention of the audience is needed in addition to a shared platform of concepts.

Is (ii) a condition that is relevant in both face-to-face and interactive communication in the way (i) is? It is since speakers always need the attention of their audience in order to be able to communicate beliefs and thoughts. The differences between the two forms of communication do not matter; (ii) represents a fundamental communicative aim both in face-to-face and in interactive communication.

At the same time there is an obvious difference between face-to-face and interactive communication: it is much easier to secure the attention of an audience in the former than in the latter. After all, speakers are normally able to see whether they have the attention of their audience, and it is also easier for them to understand how to proceed in order to secure attention. Again, this does not apply without exception. Audiences might ostensibly understand and internalize what a speaker says but nevertheless make it clear later that they have not formed the beliefs that speakers intend to communicate. Causes can be states of shock or stress but also, less dramatically, lack of genuine attention or problems of concentration.

It is equally evident that the third communication condition that focused on associate misunderstandings applies in both face-to-face and interactive communication. Both forms of communication can involve audiences who associate a message with beliefs and thoughts that are radically different from the beliefs and thoughts that a speaker has. Whether or not the communicators observe each other is not crucial for this. An audience who hears a speaker over the phone might ascribe to the speaker beliefs that the speaker does not have, even though the audience understands what is literally expressed by the sentence in question, as the above 'The ambulance is on its way' case clearly illustrated. But this case could also be redescribed to show how a similar misunderstanding could occur face-to-face.

Imagine for instance a doctor who tells a patient who has been hospitalized for some time that 'Your condition has really improved'. The patient takes this to mean that the doctor thinks that he will be able to leave the hospital within a few days, he becomes frustrated when this turn out to not happen, and we might even imagine that he tells relatives that the doctor gave him false expectations. The problem, we may assume, is that the doctor does not associate the belief that the patient's condition has improved with the belief that the patient should be sent home within a few days. He does not mean to commit himself to this or any other specific interpretation of 'improved condition'.[7]

Even though these two cases clearly show that associate misunderstandings can occur both in face-to-face and interactive interaction, they also suggest an argument for the view that they more often occur in the former than the latter. When doctors in situations like the above utter sentences like 'Your condition has really improved', it is not unusual for patients to ask 'Does this mean that I will be able to go home soon?' if they are concerned about this. There is typically more of an atmosphere of dialogue and conversation in face-to-face communication, and this often causes audiences to clarify their own perspectives and make inquires about the speaker's beliefs. In fact, communicators' overall communicative aim is often to clarify their own perspectives and the perspectives of the persons they are talking

---

[7] This kind of misunderstanding is sometimes displayed in newspapers, under headlines like 'The doctor gave me six months to live'. One should be sceptical about the idea that doctors very often state predictions in such a bold way. In fact, what has often been stated is something much weaker ('There is a significant possibility that...'), but patients often associate these statements with stronger claims. This is a general phenomenon that most professionals involved in interaction with various forms of clients or patients should be aware of: we tend to forget qualifications like 'significant possibility' after a while, and we think of claims that have been made as much stronger than what they in reality were.

to. Associate misunderstandings typically occur when the situation is hectic, or when there is for some other reason poor dialogue about different aspects of the issue of discourse. In interactive communication, the problem is often that it takes a lot of time to clarify one's own perspective extensively.

The same point applies in connection with the last communication condition (iv), which focused on incorrect ascriptions of experiences and values, but now communicators face an additional challenge that makes observation even more significant. On the phone or via radio a person's subjective states can only be presented as descriptions or single words that express these states. Everything depends on the interpretation that the audience makes; the language that is heard on the phone or seen on the screen is the only interpretative clue. An observable communicative context, on the other hand, will often provide vital clues to the nature of an underlying experience. An adequate understanding of a pain state will normally be easier to achieve in face-to-face encounters because a person's body language tends to reveal intrinsic aspects of the state.

As long as a person's immediate surroundings provide important clues to his social and cultural background a similar point applies when values are communicated. Our personal values, the activities we like to participate in and the complex ways we wish to live our lives, are first and foremost accessible by observations of how we actually choose to live our lives in the contexts we are in. In this sense similarities and differences in values are often easier to detect face-to-face than interactively, and incorrect attributions of values do not occur so easily.

There is a further even more fundamental difference between the fourth and the first three communication conditions. The first three focus on conditions for communication of concept-involving propositional attitudes like beliefs and thoughts. This means that they are subject to the aim of understanding as a 'fusion of horizon', the idea that fundamental understanding is a matter of speaker and audience sharing subjective states involving the same concepts (Gadamer 1975, 1994; Mueller-Vollmer 1986; Green 2000). A speaker and an audience who share many of the same beliefs have cognitive horizons that are much more similar than communicators who do not have many of the same beliefs. From the perspective of a speaker, the practical implications of this idea that a fusion of horizons should be regarded as an aim of understanding can be formulated as three action-guiding questions. Corresponding to the first communication condition (i), does the audience have an understanding of the language I use that is sufficiently similar to my own understanding? Corresponding to the second condition (ii), do I have the genuine attention of the audience? And corresponding to the third (iii), is it reasonable to think that the audience will associate the belief that I express literally in language with other beliefs that are radically different from the beliefs I have?

It is important to recognize that since the fourth condition does not focus on conceptual states a similar question related to the idea of a shared horizon cannot be formulated. An experiential state like pain does not involve concepts that can be shared with another person. Of course, if a person reports 'I am in pain', and if an interpreter takes this to mean that the person is in pain, then they share the concept *pain*. But as emphasized above, this is not the same as sharing the state of pain. Similarly with values; a speaker might appreciate living his life in a certain way and attempt to communicate this value to an audience by using a particular sentence. The audience might associate this sentence with the same concepts as the speaker, but this does not mean that they share the same value. In order to understand what the underlying value is, the audience needs to take a further step and identify the value state that lies beneath the surface of language. A misunderstanding of the fourth kind occurs when this attempt fails. The question a speaker needs to ask in order to prevent misunderstandings of this kind is therefore this: have I correctly understood the values of my audience, and is there a chance that I will be ascribed values that I do not have?

This question about values should be sharply distinguished from the question of whether a person expresses a true or false subjective state. A belief is subject to rational discussion about truth and falsity;

if someone thinks that a person has a false belief, he can rationally try to show the person that the proposition he believes in is false. Since values are attitudes to activities and not propositions, they are not subject to similar questions about objectivity. If someone wants to influence or change another person's values, the only rational way of doing so is to go beneath them, to locate possible beliefs and thoughts they are grounded in. For instance, I appreciate drinking a lot of coffee. This is an everyday personal value I have, but I would not have it if I formed the belief that drinking a lot of coffee is very unhealthy. So, if a person I consider to be a medical expert explained to me that me my activity is very unhealthy, then I would probably form this belief, and I would no longer have my value.

It is therefore sometimes possible to change a person's values by identifying unjustified beliefs that support them. The problem arises only if we think that a person's values are equivalent to beliefs and thoughts and consequently attempts to show the person that his values are not 'objectively correct'. A person who is subject to such a criticism will typically feel that we are encroaching on a private sphere that we are not entitled to enter; the person has already an implicit grasp of the nature of personal values as subjective states that we have an individual right to form.

A further discussion of this issue would fall outside the scope of this chapter, but I think it has been important to make it clear exactly why successful communication presupposes that communicators, implicitly or explicitly, are able to distinguish beliefs and thoughts from personal values. A fundamental identification of a person's values is often crucial for successful communication, regardless whether or not we want to change these values.

7. Conclusion

By using examples from paramedic-patient interaction within a theoretical framework from philosophy of mind and language, I have tried to explain how the idea of communication conditions can be used to analyze communication. In doing so I have made a distinction between four fundamental conditions. The first focuses on the idea of a shared language, the second on communicative attention, the third on the way we associate beliefs with other beliefs, and the fourth on subjective states like experiences and values that do not have a conceptual, propositional content.

I have argued that these four conditions constitute fundamental communicative aims both face-to-face and in interactive communication. At the same time they suggest different strategies for how these aims should be achieved within the two realms of communication. The fact that the four conditions cover both forms of communication constitutes a fundamental justification for adopting these strategies in face-to-face and interactive interaction. This does not mean that the conditions imply that it is easier to secure successful face-to-face communication than it is to secure interactive communication. Obviously, it is natural to assume that it is often easier to achieve the former than the latter (there are some obvious exceptions), but the question of whether this really is so remains a further question. My aim has been to develop a plausible framework for addressing this and other normative questions related to face-to-face and interactive communication.

In addition to this instrumental justification for applying the communication conditions, I think it is important to recognize a further argument. It is sometimes held that an instrumental justification of a theory must be essentially incomplete, since it is possible for an instrumental theory to be false (Dennett 1978). But in this context I do not think this is a genuine possibility. Philosophical theories of communication are after all meant to capture ordinary discourse – it is standardly assumed that whether they do or not is what makes them true or false – so in this case the fact that the conditions match our communicative practices constitutes a good reason for holding that they are true. Too often philosophical theories of communication are developed in isolation from areas of application, even though it is claimed that they are grounded in common sense. What I have tried to show is that the four communication conditions are really grounded in ordinary communicative practices.

Finally, I would like to make it clear that it has not been possible to discuss in detail the practical consequences of the analyses I have made within the limits here. The aim has been to develop and clarify some fundamental philosophical distinctions and to point out some reasonable implications of these distinctions. However, more empirical research is necessary to explore these implications further. What I have offered is a framework for doing such research, but this is a framework that in it self should be modified and developed further on the basis of research.

References

Bechtel W and Graham G (1998). *A companion to cognitive science*. Oxford: Blackwell publishing.

Bezuidenhout A (1997). 'The Communication of de re thoughts'. *NOUS*, 31, 197–225.

Burge T (1979). 'Individualism and the Mental'. *Midwest studies in philosophy*, 4, 73–120.

Burge T (1989). 'Wherein is Language Social?' In: A. George (ed): *Reflections on Chomsky*. Oxford: Blackwell.

Cappelen H and Lepore E (2005). *Insensitive semantics*. Oxford: Blackwell publishing.

Dancy J (1996). *Moral reasons*. Oxford: Blackwell publishing.

Davies M. (1995). 'Philosophy of mind'. In: A C Grayling (ed): *Philosophy: A guide through the subject*. Oxford: Oxford University Press.

Davies M (1998). 'Externalism, architecturalism, and epistemic warrant'. In: C. Wright, B. Smith and C. Macdonald (eds): *Knowing our own minds*. Oxford: Oxford University Press.

Davidson D (1984). *Inquires into truth and interpretation*. Oxford: Clarendon Press.

Davidson D (1987). 'Knowing one's own mind', *Proceedings of the American philosophical association*, 61, 430–70.

Dennett D (1978). *Consciousness explained*. Middlesex: Penguin Books.

Eide T and Eide H (2004). *Kommunikasjon i praksis*. Oslo: Gyldendal akademisk.

Enelow A, Forde D and Brummel-Smith K (1996). *Interviewing and patient care*. Oxford: Oxford University Press.

Gadamer H G (1975). *Truth and method*. New York: Seabury Press

Gadamer H G (1994). *Literature and philosophy in dialogue*. Albany NY: State University of New York Press.

Green G (2000). *Theology, hermeneutics, and imagination: The crisis of interpretation at the end of modernity*. Cambridge: Cambridge University Press.

Guttenplan S (1996). *A companion to philosophy of mind*. Oxford: Blackwell publishing.

Johnston P (1989). *Wittgenstein and moral philosophy*. London: Routledge.

Kripke S (1982). *Wittgenstein on rules and private language*. Oxford: Blackwell publishing.

Mechanic D (1968). *Medical sociology*. New York/London: The Free Press.

Mueller-Vollmer K (1986). *The hermeneutics reader: Texts of the German tradition from the enlightenment to the present*. Oxford: Blackwell publishing.

Nettleton S (1995). *The sociology of health and illness*. Cambridge UK: Polity Press.

Nordby H (2004a). 'The importance of knowing how to talk about illness without applying the concept of illness'. *Nursing philosophy*, 5, 30–40.

Nordby H (2004b). 'Communicative challenges for paramedics'. *Scandinavian journal of trauma, resuscitation and emergency medicine*, 12, 178–182.

Nordby H (2004c). 'Incorrect understanding and concept possession'. *Philosophical explorations*, 7, 51–75.

Nordby H (2006). 'Nurse-patient-interaction: Language mastery and concept possession'. *Nursing inquiry*, 13, 64–72.

Peacocke C (1992). *A study of concepts*. Cambridge MA: MIT Press.

Peacocke C (1998). *Being known*. Oxford: Clarendon Press.

Pessin A and Goldberg S (1996). *The twin earth chronicles*. New York/London: M.E. Sharpe.

Putnam H (1981). *Reason, truth and history*. Cambridge: Cambridge University Press.

Radley A (1994). *Making sense of illness*. London: Sage publications.

Rosenthal D (1991). *The nature of mind*. Oxford: Oxford University Press.

Ryle G (1949). *The concept of mind*. London: Huchinson.

Smith N (1997). *Strong hermeneutics: Contingency and moral identity* London: Routledge.

Tjora A (1997). *Caring machines*. Dr. polit thesis in sociology. Trondheim: NTNU.

Travelbee J (1971). *Interpersonal aspects of nursing*. Philadelphia: Davis.

Warnke G (1987). *Gadamer: Hermeneutics, tradition, and reason*. Stanford CA: Stanford University Press.

Wittgenstein L (1953). *Philosophical investigations*. Oxford: Blackwell publishing.

Worhall J and Worhall J (2003). 'Defining disease: Much ado about nothing?' *Analecta husserliana*, 72, 33–55.

Chapter 4

The analytic-synthetic distinction and conceptual analyses of basic health concepts

Summary Within philosophy of medicine it has been a widespread view that there are important theoretical and practical reasons for clarifying the nature of basic health concepts like *disease, illness* and *sickness*. Many theorists have attempted to give definitions that can function as general standards, but as more and more definitions have been rejected as inadequate, pessimism about the possibility of formulating plausible definitions has become increasingly widespread. However, the belief that no definitions will succeed since no definitions have succeeded is an inductive objection, open to realist responses. The chapter argues that an influential argument from philosophy of language constitutes a more fundamental objection. I use *disease* as an example and show that this argument implies that if a common understanding of *disease* can be analysed into a definition, then this is a non-trivial definition. But any non-trivial analysis must be viciously circular: the analysis must presuppose that *disease* can be defined, but this is what the analysis is supposed to yield as a result. This means, the chapter concludes, that *disease* and other controversial health concepts do not have analyses grounded in a common language. Stipulative and contextual definitions can have local significance, but the normative roles of such definitions are at the same time limited.

1. Introduction

In philosophy of medicine, many attempts have been made to give a more precise definition of basic health concepts like *health*, *disease*, *illness* and *sickness*. The significance of these attempts has first and foremost been linked to the concepts' normative roles. It has been thought that questions concerning the application of the concepts are important within many areas of health care and health policy, and that definitions of the concepts can constitute standards for how they should be applied (Albert, Munson and Resnik 1988; Nordenfelt 1987, 2001; Nordenfelt and Twaddle 1993). The traditional strategy for achieving this normative aim has been to base the definitions in ordinary language. The reason, as Nordenfelt (1987, 8) says, is that an analysis that does not capture a common understanding 'would not be used in ordinary discourse, and would therefore be of no interest to us'.

The concept *disease* is probably the health concept that has been subject to most conceptual analyses, but despite many attempts to formulate a general definition of disease none has received widespread acceptance (Worhall and Worhall 2001; Hofmann 2001). One possible explanation is that the definition of *disease* really exists, but that it is difficult to find this definition. This realism about the existence of a definition implies that one should, at least in principle, continue to search for the definition (Burge 1990; Peacocke 1998). A more pessimistic explanation is that there is no definition to be found. According to this sceptical view, there is no fact of the matter to disagree about in this area.

The sceptical view has gained proponents in recent years as an increasing number of analyses of *disease* have been claimed to fail. Worhall and Worhall (2001, 55) claim that the project of defining *disease* is a 'degenerative project', that 'there is no reason to think that any such adequate general characterisation of disease can be developed'. Hofmann (2001, 230) has in a similar spirit claimed that the diversity of analyses suggests that a 'simple definition of disease cannot be obtained'.[8]

These arguments use the controversy surrounding the nature of *disease* as evidence for the general conclusion that the concept cannot be defined. In this sense the arguments are inductive, and it is important to remember that the power of the arguments is therefore limited. It is true that the controversy supports the sceptical view, but one makes an unjustified argumentative leap if one in addition claims that the controversy implies that the concept cannot be defined (Burge 1990). If one wants to give more than an inductive argument, what is needed is an argument grounded in philosophy of language. The argument must show that our common English concept has a content that cannot be captured in a definition.

The aim of this chapter is to present such an argument. In the next two sections I clarify the potential significance and normative aim of attempts to analyse basic health concepts like *disease*. I then present evaluative and naturalistic definitions of *disease* and argue that discussions of these definitions have not paid attention to an important philosophical argument. According to this argument, the attempt to define a common understanding is equivalent to formulating a definition that is analytic in the sense that it is true 'in virtue of meaning'. But like Quine (1953, 1969, 1985) I argue that no such definition can be formulated: conceptual analysis of *disease* cannot yield a pure conceptual truth about our common concept. This conclusion, I maintain, generalises to all attempts to make conceptual analyses of basic health concepts: it is impossible to formulate definitions of concepts like *health*, *illness* and *sickness* that are grounded in our common language.

In the last part of the chapter I discuss implications of this argument. I argue that poor communication can be reduced if participants in

---

[8] Uffe Juel Jensen (1983) is a third example. He has claimed that a definition of disease is unable to incorporate the fact that the concept is an ever-changing, ever-evolving concept. However, Juel Jensen's arguments are inconclusive. Why should the contention that no definition has managed to capture the concept so far imply that it is impossible for a definition to do so?

medical discourse do not presuppose that controversial health concepts have general definitions. The argument is at the same time consistent with the idea that the concepts have important contextual and stipulative normativity within different areas. Like Nordenfelt (1993) I distinguish between four areas that deserve special attention: the philosophy of welfare, the health care setting, the clinical context and the medical sciences. Furthermore, contextual meaning-explanations and idiosyncratic conceptions of disease and illness can play important roles in interaction between speakers who do not understand the concepts in the same way.

2. Background – normativity and grey cases

The question of the nature of basic health concepts like *disease*, *illness* and *sickness* should be distinguished from the question of why it is important to discuss the nature of these concepts. The main focus of this chapter is the first question, but in order to clarify its significance it is necessary first to say something about the second. In order to have a clear focus I will in the following focus mostly on *disease*, since this is the concept that has received most attention. After having made it clear how the argument I will develop applies in the case of *disease*, I will show how it applies to conceptual analyses of health concepts in general.

In their influential *Reasoning in Medicine* (1988) Albert, Munson and Resnik present three reasons why it is important to clarify *disease*. Firstly, they hold (1988, 150) that the 'disease concept is a central notion in medicine, and that, in itself, makes it worthy of attention'. In particular, a proper understanding of the role of the concept in medical practice 'requires that we understand the meaning of the concept as it is actually employed in clinical medicine' (150). Secondly, the application of the concept within medicine has important consequences for other parts of society. For instance, 'if excessive drinking, unruliness in children, or a tendency to act violently are diseases or symptoms of diseases, then medicine has an implicit mandate to eliminate them'

(151). Thirdly, different forms of disease can only be classified on the basis of assumptions about disease in general. If such classifications are to be 'conducted in accordance with nonarbitrary principles, then we must make explicit the assumptions about the nature of disease that are employed in those activities' (152).

As Albert, Munson and Resnik observe, these reasons for discussing the nature of *disease* can be explored in different ways. They acknowledge, moreover, that there can be further reasons for elucidating the concept. Their point is that in order to establish that it is important to shed light on the nature of *disease,* 'these three are sufficiently important to make it unnecessary to cast about for others' (150).

It should be emphasised that the assumption that it is important to elucidate the nature of *disease* does not imply that it is possible to state a general definition; it is possible to hold that an analysis is needed and at the same time maintain that it does not have to be a definition. This point is not always stated clearly in the literature. Hofmann aims to capture the traditional view when he writes that

> [w]e need a concept of disease in order to decide who is entitled to treatment and to economic rights, who is to be exempted from social duties and who is morally accountable, and to decide what is the subject matter of medical science. Furthermore, a strictly, consistently and coherently defined concept of disease could help the health care system face its basic economical, social, epistemological and ethical challenges, and could clarify the goal and limit of medicine (Hofmann 2001, 211).

One should distinguish between two claims Hofmann makes. Firstly, there is the claim that medicine actually needs a proper definition of *disease*. This, in turn, is consistent with various views about the exact role and importance of the definition. Some theorists have focused on clinical practice while others have focused on broader issues within health policy. Furthermore, there has been disagreement about the role of the definition with respect to other basic health concepts. Some have argued that insight into the application conditions of *disease* can be gained independently of analyses of *illness* and *sickness*, while others have argued that *disease* cannot be analysed independently of these concepts (Hofmann 2002; Nordenfelt and Twaddle 1993).

Hofmann's second claim, that a definition of *disease* could help the health care system, is weaker than the first. In order to accept this second claim it is sufficient that one thinks that if a proper definition can be formulated, then that definition should be used to meet fundamental challenges within medicine. Accepting this is consistent with holding that the same challenges can be met in other ways, not necessarily on the basis of a general definition.

For the present argumentative purposes it is not important to choose between these views. The important point is that all the parties in the traditional debate have accepted that it is important to clarify the nature of *disease*. Consequently, *if* it is possible to define *disease*, then that has important intrinsic and extrinsic consequences for medicine. This conditional, I will assume here, constitutes the fundamental motivation for exploring whether the concept can be defined.

Within this framework, the nature of *disease* has often been discussed in connection with what one has thought of as grey cases of disease. The idea has been as follows: the concept applies to a number of bodily states a person can be in. AIDS, cancer, myocardial infarction, measles, tuberculosis and diabetes are uncontroversial cases. It is equally clear that the concept does not apply to many states a person can be in, even states that can affect well-being or normal functioning. Qualitative states like headache, tiredness or stiffness are sometimes not regarded as disease or symptoms of disease. The same applies to many physical states that are not always accompanied by qualitative states. Suffering from a scratch or a minor injury is not having a disease.

In addition to the clear cases, there are cases of uncertainty or disagreement. Many mental illnesses have been thought of as such 'grey cases'. Other controversial cases are fibromyalgia, whiplash, lower back pain and chronic fatigue syndrome. Many grey cases arise from a long lasting negative experience, like the experience of pain, where the medical profession has been unable to identify an underlying physical cause.

The fundamental motivation for analysing *disease* has been the need for arriving at reasonable verdicts about the grey cases (Worhall and Worhall 2001). One can imagine a doctor who tells a patient that it has not been possible to locate an underlying physical cause of the pain the patient has experienced in his neck for a long time. The patient asks if this means that he does not have a disease. For the patient it is important to know whether the label 'disease' applies to him. The doctor, however, finds it difficult to give him the yes-or-no answer the patient desires. The hope has been that a careful conceptual analysis of the concept of disease can clarify its conceptual content so that it becomes clearer to the medical profession how grey cases should be judged:

> Perhaps philosophers, with their expertise in conceptual matters, can provide significant help here by providing a clear-cut and defensible characterisation, not of any particular disease (that seems clearly a scientific issue), but of the class of diseases – of what might be called 'disease-in-general' (Worhall and Worhall 2001, 33).

What must a characterisation of disease look like in order to meet this challenge? An account that merely gives necessary applications will yield an answer only in cases where these conditions are not met (the concept does not apply). The same problem of incompleteness faces analyses that merely give sufficient conditions. Such analyses yield an answer only when these conditions are present (the concept applies). The aim has therefore been to give both necessary and sufficient conditions. Such a characterisation would not only be of help in a limited set of grey cases, but it would have normative implications in general. Giving such a characterisation, it will be assumed here, is giving a definition of disease.[9]

3. Conceptual analysis

For the argumentative purposes of this chapter it is important to understand how the project of analysing basic health concepts like *disease* falls under the general idea of conceptual analysis. Harman has formulated the general idea of conceptual analysis in an illuminating way:

> Typically, attempts at philosophical analysis proceed by the formulation of one or more tentative analyses and then the consideration of test cases. If exactly one of the proposed analyses does not conflict with 'intuitions' about any test cases, it is taken to be at least tentatively confirmed. Further research then uncovers new test cases in which intuitions conflict with the analysis. The analysis is then modified or replaced by a completely different one, which is in turn tested against imagined cases, and so on (Harman 1999, 139).

A conceptual analysis can implement this procedure in different ways, but as Harman points out, all conceptual analyses share some

---

[9] Some theorists have seemed to think that those who have attempted to define *disease* have failed to recognise that the concept has dimensions that cannot be captured in a definition (Lupton 1994). But the traditional motivation for defining *disease* has not been the idea that only a definition can elucidate important aspects of the concept. The motivation has been that only a definition can have general normative implications. It is consistent with this view to hold that there are aspects of the concept that it is important to clarify, even though they cannot be captured in a definition.

substantive assumptions.[10] One is that there is a definition of the target concept to be found. This, moreover, should not merely reflect a special understanding or be a stipulative definition (Quine 1953; 1960). A stipulative definition can be useful within the context it is restricted to, but it does not constitute a general normative standard. In philosophy of medicine, what one has sought to find is a definition of *disease* that captures a common understanding. The hope has been that if such a definition can be articulated, then participants in medical discourse, both laymen and professionals, will defer to this articulation since it matches their implicit understanding of the word 'disease'.

Lennart Nordenfelt is perhaps the theorist who has expressed this idea most clearly, in his discussion of the concept of health. While a study of how people understand this concept is a descriptive study, Nordenfelt claims that

> [...] the present project is more traditionally philosophical; its purpose is to find a core element in prevalent uses of the term 'health', and try to develop it in such ways that it will become coherent and useful for scientific purposes. The aim is not merely one of lexicography, but also of logical reconstruction: to sharpen the borders of the concept of health. The concept will thus be influenced by the process of analysis (Nordenfelt 1987, 11).

This means that the 'scientific and coherent' concept the analysis is searching for can be found only if the concept has 'fairy clear

---

[10] This is important, since some might think that there is something fundamentally wrong with conceptual analysis in general. It might be held, for instance, that any conceptual analysis requires that intuitions can be separated from theory. This objection is implausible since it is possible to hold that a person's intuitions cannot be separated from the rest of his beliefs, but that his intuitions nevertheless are important for evaluating test cases. Such a position is similar to empirical holism, the view that empirical statements have a special role in confirmation of an empirical theory, even though they form a part of the overall theory (Quine 1953).

boundaries and that these can be detected by a careful analysis' (Nordenfelt 1987, 9).

Attempts to define *disease* have had the same goal (Engelhardt 1975; Campell et al. 1979; Resnek 1987; Nordenfelt and Twaddle 1993; Humber and Almeder 1997; Worhall and Worhall 2001; Hofmann 2001; 2002). The starting point has been the desire to arrive at a reasonable verdict about grey cases, and in trying to achieve this aim one has attempted to develop an account of disease that meets the following conditions: (1) The account is a definition, (2) the account captures a common understanding, and (3) the account (therefore) gives a reasonable verdict about grey cases. This threefold normativity condition sums up the traditional aim of conceptual analysis of *disease*. The idea has been that an account that meets conditions (1)–(3) has met an overall condition for being a correct articulation of our common concept.

4. Attempts to define disease

In this section I present central aspects of the traditional debate on the nature of *disease*. The aim is to show that the problems that have been identified do not really show that the concept cannot be defined. I will argue that in order to establish the sceptical conclusion one needs an argument that focuses comprehensively on the project of making conceptual analysis of *disease*.

Attempts to define *disease* have traditionally been categorised as evaluative and naturalistic strategies. An evaluative strategy seeks to define *disease* partly or wholly in evaluative terms, by appealing to the evaluative judgements a person or group of persons would make involving the concept. This framework is similar to frameworks that have commonly been used to analyse *sickness* and *illness*. Having a sickness, it is often held, is to be judged by the community as having a certain role (Marinker 1975; Nordenfelt and Twaddle 1993). Illness, on the other hand, is supposed to reflect experiences from a first-person perspective. Correspondingly, it has been suggested that *disease* reflects a third perspective, namely the perspective of the medical profession. Hofmann has presented such a view when he suggests that

> Disease is negative bodily occurrences as conceived of by the medical profession. Illness is negative bodily occurrences as conceived of by the person himself. Correspondingly, sickness is negative bodily occurrence as conceived of by the society and/ or its institutions (Hofmann 2002, 150).

Hofmann thinks of this as an account and not a definition, but he argues that the account nevertheless has useful normative implications. I will not discuss these arguments here. What I want to focus on is whether the account – definition or not – can meet the above normativity condition.

One initial problem is connected to the idea of a medical profession. Who are to be counted as members of the medical profession (Freidson 1988)? Note also that the account cannot solve the problem of grey cases. If there is agreement among members of the medical profession about a case, then the case is hardly a grey case. But if there is uncertainty or disagreement in the medical profession about a grey case, then it follows from the above account that the problem of the application of *disease* remains unsolved.

A second problem that confronts an evaluative strategy is that one can end up with wrong verdicts about some clearly negative cases. During the 19th century it was common to regard homosexuality as a disease. Not only would we strongly deny that it is a disease today, we would also deny that it was a disease then (Hofmann 2002). A similar problem confronts Scadding's definition. He suggests that a disease is 'the sum of the abnormal phenomena displayed by a group of living organisms in association with a specified [...] set of characteristics by which they differ from the norm for their species' (Scadding 1967, 25). Again, as long as the definition relies on 'our norms' at a given time, then one faces the problem of explaining who 'we' are, and the problem that 'we' might be wrong.

A third initial problem for an evaluative strategy is even more directly connected to the assumption that the definition should constitute a normative standard. Imagine a given grey case: is this a disease or not? All that an evaluative definition can tell us is that in order to answer this we have to address a further issue, namely the issue of what the evaluations of some group of persons would be. The problem of giving the correct judgement is merely shifted back to the problem of explaining who one should turn to (Worhall and Worhall 2001).

It is reasonable to suppose that it is recognition of these obvious problems that explains why the majority of definitions of *disease* have sought to apply naturalistic terms. There is no commonly accepted definition of what a naturalistic term is, but the guiding rule has been that a term is naturalistic if and only if it is used in explanations in the natural sciences (Guttenplan 1996). This understanding is sufficiently precise here.

One of the classical naturalistic analyses of *disease* is Marinker's suggestion that disease is a 'pathological process most often physical as in throat infection, a cancer of the bronchus, sometimes undetermined in origin, as in schizophrenia. The quality which identifies disease is some deviation from a biological norm' (Marinker 1975, 81). An initial problem with this suggestion is that imprecise terms like 'most often' and 'sometimes' are inadequate in a proper definition. Similarly, it is unclear what a 'biological norm' is. What is regarded as a plausible description of a biological norm at one time might later be thought of as inadequate.

Another well-known attempt to define *disease* is Boorse's definition of *disease* as a type 'of internal state which is either an impairment of normal functional ability, i.e. a reduction of one or more functional abilities below typical efficiency, or a limitation on functional ability caused by environmental agents' (Boorse 1997, 8–9). Boorse's definition has been criticised for being circular and for being imprecise. It has also been criticised for excluding states that should be included and for including states that should be excluded. In particular, and as Worhall and Worhall (2001, 45) observe, the 'clause about "limitation on functional ability caused by environmental agents" threatens, for example, to make being held in gaol count as a disease'. Boorse, in fact, accepts that his definition is one among several possible definitions of disease. One might think that this is an insignificant move, but it is, in fact, a move that changes the project completely. For now one faces the question: which definition should be applied in cases of disagreement or uncertainty? None of the definitions would function as *the* normative standard.

The problem of lack of clarity and the problem of normativity need to be addressed by attempts to define *disease*, but it is not given *a priori* that they cannot be solved. On the contrary, a semantic realist will insist that they can be solved. He thinks that the concept has a real determinate extension, and that there must be some way of describing this extension in a definition. The fact that no definition has so far received widespread acceptance merely shows, according to the semantic realist, that it is difficult to uncover the correct definition (Burge 1990; Peacocke 1998).

A convincing objection to the idea that the concept of disease can be defined needs to address this realism about the existence of a definition; it must show that the idea that the concept has a determinate extension is false. The objection must therefore be grounded in philosophy of language, in considerations about the status of the conceptual content of the concept *disease*.

In the following I will begin to develop such an objection, and a dialogue between Twaddle and Nordenfelt can serve as a starting point. Twaddle has defined disease as 'a health problem that consists of a physiological malfunction that results in an actual or potential reduction in physical capacities and/or reduced life expectancy' (Nordenfelt and Twaddle 1993, 8). Nordenfelt comments that this makes injuries, impairments and other bodily defects instances of disease, and he suggests that these states should instead be thought of as useful additions to the concept of disease. Twaddle responds that he perhaps 'is more inclusive of events under the concept of disease than is Nordenfelt' (Nordenfelt and Twaddle 1993, 41).

Twaddle's willingness to let the definition of disease have a wider scope than what Nordenfelt thinks appropriate poses a challenge for someone who thinks that a general definition can be formulated. For if participants in the debate disagree about what states should fall under the definition, then they will necessarily end up with different definitions. The dialogue between Nordenfelt and Twaddle seem to constitute a good reason for reflecting further on the idea that a general definition can be derived from a common understanding.

5. The analytic-synthetic argument

To someone acquainted with modern philosophy of language it might seem somewhat curious that discussions of the nature of *disease* have not paid more attention to an influential philosophical argument. According to this argument, it is impossible to define concepts in the way one has attempted to analyse *disease*. Any such attempt, the argument holds, must either be question-begging or viciously circular. This means that the traditional discussions of the challenges that confront evaluative and naturalistic definitions in the end are insignificant; the philosophical argument will imply that it impossible in principle to define *disease*.

The analytic-synthetic argument, as it has often been labelled, is primarily associated with Willard Quine (1960; 1969), but it has been formulated and discussed by a number of philosophers (Putnam 1962; Davidson 1984; Fodor 1987; Guttenplan 1996). The argument consists of two argumentative steps. The first step claims that (1) no concept definitions are obviously analytic. The term 'analytic' is here thought of as 'true purely in virtue of meaning' (and sentences that are not 'true in virtue of meaning' are 'synthetic'). The condition for being true in virtue of meaning is, in turn, connected to understanding: if a sentence is true purely in virtue of meaning, then anyone who understands it understands that it is true. Consequently, a sentence is obviously analytic if and only if anyone who understands it realises that it is true.

On the basis of this conception of analycity, the idea behind (1) can be explained as follows: to understand what a sentence means is to understand what the involved words mean. To understand what the sentence 'Arthritis causes stiffness' means is to understand that 'arthritis' means *arthritis*, that 'causes' means *causes*, and that 'stiffness' means *stiffness*. In other words, understanding the sentence involves possession of the three concepts that the words express. If the sentence is obviously analytic, then anyone who is able to think the thought *arthritis causes stiffness* realises that this thought is true (Harman 1999).

It should be emphasised that (1) is consistent with the idea that some sentences are obviously analytic. It is plausible to assume that anyone who is able to think the thought that arthritis is a disease or arthritis is not a disease understands that this thought is true. It is impossible to think this thought and genuinely believe that it is false. But the reason it is true is that it is a logical truth that X is p or X is not p: 'In general a logical truth is a statement which is true and remains true under all reinterpretations of its components other than the logical particles' (Quine 1985, 27).

However, (1) does not claim that there are no analytic sentences. What (1) claims is that it is impossible to give definitions of concepts that are obviously analytic. A classical example of a concept definition that has been thought of as analytic is 'A bachelor is an unmarried man'. As Quine observes, the idea has been that this sentence is obviously analytic since 'it can be turned into a logical truth by putting synonyms for synonyms [...] by putting "unmarried man" for its synonym "bachelor." The problem, according to Quine, is that 'we still lack a proper characterisation of this second class of analytic statements' (Quine 1985, 32).

According to the suggestion the analytic-synthetic argument is targeted at, the concept *bachelor* can uncontroversially be defined as *unmarried man*. But Quine claims that it is not obviously true that a person is a bachelor if and only if he is an unmarried man; it is not the case that everyone who possesses the concept *bachelor* thinks that a bachelor has to be unmarried. According to Quine, even the most plausible candidates for being analytic are, in reality, vulnerable to doubt. In a recent exposition of the analytic-synthetic argument, Harman states this point in an illuminating way:

> When Quine, Putnam, Winograd and a host of others raised objections to the analytic-synthetic distinction, they did not mention controversial philosophical analyses. When problems were raised about particular conceptual claims, they were problems about the examples that had been offered as seemingly clear cases [...] [like] 'Unmarried adult male humans are bachelors' and 'Women are female' [...] People will not apply the term 'bachelor' to a man who lives with the same woman over a long enough period of time even if they are not married. Society pages in newspapers will identify as eligible 'bachelors' men who are in the process of being divorced but are still married. The Olympic Committee may have rejected certain women as insufficiently female on the basis of their chromosomes (Harman 1999, 140).

The same point applies to *disease* and other medical concepts. The sentence 'Arthritis is inflammation of the joints' might seem to be true in virtue of meaning. But in order for the sentence to qualify as obviously analytic everybody who is capable of thinking that arthritis is inflammation of the joints must realise that the thought is true. However, there is widespread agreement that one does not have to understand a concept in one specific way in order to possess it. One does not have to have expert knowledge of the application condition of the concept *arthritis* in order to possess it. For a medical layman, the thought that arthritis is inflammation of the joints does not have to be an obvious truth (Putnam 1975; Burge 1979).

The first step of the analytic-synthetic argument is a generalisation of this point: definitions of concepts might have an immediate appeal to those who have a complete understanding of the concept involved, but the definitions do not meet the overall condition for being obviously analytic.

What if one, instead of trying to find obvious truths, attempted to show that some concept definitions are analytic? The second step of the analytic-synthetic argument is a response to this suggestion. It claims that (2) any argument that seeks to establish that a sentence is analytic must be viciously circular.

The idea behind (2) is as follows: suppose that one tried to formulate a convincing argument for the view that *disease* can be defined as 'negative bodily occurrences as conceived of by the medical profession', in accordance with Hofmann's above account. Note that in order for such an argument to be sound, it cannot contain as a premise the claim that *disease* has the extension specified by this definition. For this claim is what the argument is supposed to yield as a conclusion. The resources that are available in a non-circular argument have, in effect, two other sources: firstly, the premises can make assumptions about the extension of the phrase that constitutes the definiens. For instance, it is possible for the argument to presuppose knowledge of what 'negative bodily occurrences' applies to.

Secondly, the premises of a non-circular argument can make assumptions about *disease* as long as they are not assumptions about the content of the concept. One can, for instance, make assumptions about the use of the word 'disease'. What one cannot do is make assumptions about the correct definition of *disease*. To make such invalid assumptions, I will assume, is to make normative assumptions about the concept. Thus, a convincing argument must connect descriptive facts about the concept to the claim that the concept has the correct, normative definition specified by the descriptive phrase. It must be shown that there is something about the descriptive status of the concept that establishes that the concept has the normative property of having a certain definition.

The core of Quine's analytic-synthetic argument is that this cannot be done. According to Quine, the moment one makes the inference from descriptions to a definition, then one has already made normative assumptions. Descriptive facts about *disease*, or the word 'disease' that expresses this concept, do not have normative implications. Descriptive properties tell us how the concept is actually used. A definition, on the other hand, is supposed to tell us how the concept should be used. But as Kripke (1982, 37) says, the 'relation of meaning and intention to future action is normative, not descriptive'. Facts about how *disease* is actually used do not have the required normative force.

Another formulation of the same point is that the only way to establish that two concepts are coextensional is to appeal to meaning relations between them. If I claim that descriptive fact about the use of 'disease' tells me what the extension of *disease* is, then I have already made a semantic interpretation; I have already assumed that *disease* and the definition apply to the same. Quine sums up his discussion of the attempt to reduce the meaning relation of analycity to other relations as follows:

> Analycity at first seemed most naturally definable by appeal to a realm of meanings. On refinement, the appeal to meanings gave way to an appeal to synonymy or definition. But definition turned out to be a will-o'-the-wisp, and synonymy turned out to be best understood only by dint of a prior appeal to analycity itself. So we are back at the problem of analycity (Quine 1985, 32).

Quine's point is that none of these notions can be understood independently of each other. If one has made assumptions about one of them, then one has made presuppositions about the others. Any attempt to ground a conclusion about the definition of a concept in a non-circular argument must therefore be viciously circular.

6. Implications

On the basis of this exposition of the analytic-synthetic argument, the problem confronting conceptual analyses of *disease* can be formulated as follows: the conditions that an analysis must meet are precisely the conditions that the analytic-synthetic argument claims cannot be met. If the analyses had been searching for a stipulative definition or attempted to capture a special, idiosyncratic meaning, then the analytic-synthetic argument would have no implications. But the analyses have attempted to define our common English concept and they therefore bump right into the analytic-synthetic argument. Firstly, definitions of *disease* are not logical statements but attempts to give substantive, informative content to the concept. The only option is therefore to provide some further argument for why the definition is as the analysis suggests. But it follows from the second step of the analytic-synthetic argument that any such argument must be circular. Its premises must make normative assumptions about the concept.

The application of this line of reasoning might be clearer by focusing on the above distinction between grey and clear cases. The naturalist will reason like this: there are commonly accepted applications conditions of 'disease', and we apply 'disease' if a state a person is in meets one of these conditions. We do this if we know what the condition for having diabetes is, and if we think that a person meets this condition. Furthermore, it is possible to formulate a complex disjunction that captures this and other clear cases: a state is a state of disease if it meets the condition for being diabetes, the condition for being AIDS, the condition for being cancer, and so on. This disjunction can in turn be simplified by recognising that the conditions have common elements.

One problem that confronts a proponent of this strategy is to identify exactly who are to be included among competent users of 'disease'. And for an application to count, must everyone agree, or is it sufficient that a certain percent of competent speakers agree? These are profound challenges for all attempts to analyse concepts, but as noted above, is not given in advance that the challenges cannot be met. We are too hasty if we dismiss the project of defining *disease* on these grounds. The more acute problem is that no matter how one tries to describe and systematise facts about the nature of the clear cases, these descriptions are not equivalent to a normative definition. It is the conclusion of an argument based on descriptions of the use of 'disease' that is supposed to tell us how the concept should be used. The problem lies in the inference from the descriptive facts to this conclusion.

Disease is probably the concept that has received most attention among theorists concerned with conceptual analyses of basic health concepts. I have therefore focused on this concept in the exposition of the analytic-synthetic argument, but it is easy to understand how the argument generalises. According to the analytic-synthetic argument, it is impossible to give any substantial definition of health concepts grounded in ordinary language. For instance, it is impossible to define the disputed concepts *health, illness,* and *sickness* in this way. Theorists have been interested in determining whether definitions of these concepts can be articulated, and the debate has been motivated by the need to shed light on grey cases. The idea has been that general definitions grounded in a common understanding would settle uncertainty in a way that members of our linguistic community are willing to defer to. But the analytic-synthetic argument implies that all analyses that seek to capture the ordinary meaning of *health, illness* or *sickness* must be circular.

It should be emphasised that the analytic-synthetic argument is aimed merely at attempts to define medical concepts on the basis of conceptual analyses. A large number of names and descriptions of conditions of disease and illness have been defined within medicine (Helman 1984). When confronted with these concepts, patients and other laypeople typically conceive of themselves as consumers of meaning explanations produced by members of the medical profession. Consequently, patients normally defer to the medical explanations even though they do not have an understanding that matches the content of these explanations (Burge 1979; Nettleton 1995).

The fundamental challenge that arises in discourse involving concepts like *disease* and *illness* is that these concepts have a traditional history of use outside the medical profession; it is empirically well documented that when employing these concepts patients often think they are entitled to hold on to an understanding they have learned and more or less share with other speakers in their special social and cultural contexts (Helman 1984; Lupton 1996; Nettleton 1995).

This is precisely the reason why theorists have attempted to analyse the concepts on the basis of a common understanding. But while the meaning of special medical expressions has been defined narrowly within medicine, general definitions that capture the various conceptions patients and health personnel have cannot be extracted from the diversity of understanding

7. Contextual conceptions of disease and illness

One might think that the analytic-synthetic argument implies that no attempt to define or explicate ordinary language health concepts like *health* and *disease* should be pursued. But this consequence does not follow. All the argument claims is that our common English concepts do not have definitions. This is, strictly speaking, consistent with the idea that general definitions can be developed in alternative ways. But at the same time it is important to understand how difficult this alternative project seems to be. If a definition is not grounded in a common understanding, what then is supposed to ground its general normativity?

If the alternative strategy is to succeed, then there must be some way of showing why a definition is correct even hough it does not capture a common understanding. However, remember that the aim has been to formulate definitions that both medical personnel and laypeople defer to. This requires that the definitions are conceived of as reasonable. But if a definition does not match a patient's understanding, then why should he find it reasonable to dismiss his idiosyncratic meaning and adopt an entirely new understanding?

The problem is again that the controversial concepts are controversial because they have been understood in different ways. They are, in Wittgenstein's (1953) terms, used in a variety of different 'language-games' with different implicit and explicit rules. In this terminology, the alternative strategy needs to show why one 'language-game' is more correct than others, but issues of meaning and understanding are not subject to questions of objectivity in the way issues of truth and knowledge are. Incompatible statements cannot both be true and represent knowledge at the same time, but we ordinarily accept that different speakers can understand a word in different ways. There is therefore good reason to remain sceptical to the idea that general definitions can be developed in alternative ways.

In my opinion, there is a better strategy available. The view that general definitions cannot be obtained is consistent with holding that stipulative or contextual definitions are important. Furthermore, a context of discourse need not be thought of as a restricted or highly private relation between a few speakers. If one can specify substantive assumptions about the correct use of a concept within a given area, then it should be possible to develop a definition that fit those assumptions reasonably well.

Nordenfelt has distinguished between four areas that deserve special attention. Firstly, it is important to focus on the roles that basic health concepts like *disease* and *health* have within what Nordenfelt (1993a) calls 'the philosophy of welfare': 'The health concepts are essential for our everyday understanding of the human condition: they have a central place in the political discourse concerning welfare' (Nordenfelt 1993, 17). This area, Nordenfelt, emphasises, is wider than pure philosophy of medicine insofar as its issues of focus include ethics and politics. Correspondingly, in order for definitions to be suitable for this area, they must have a nature that makes it possible to address these issues properly. These conditions that the definitions must meet are in this sense conceptual assumptions about the use of the concepts within the area.

Secondly, the health concepts play an important role in the health care setting understood as an area with an important sociological dimension: '[T]he medical enterprise and health care in general [...] influence [society] by proposing a view of the nature of health and disease to the population' (Nordenfelt 1993, 19). Crucially, by acknowledging that patients can 'legitimately abstain from work and other duties', doctors actively propose a distinction between 'the healthy and the diseased' (1993, 19). Moreover, health professionals sometimes face grey cases involving basic health concepts other than concepts associated with *disease*, like the concepts *injury*, *impairment* and *defect*. If it is possible to articulate constraints that applications of these and other disputed health concepts should meet within the health care setting, then there is a basis for developing corresponding definitions.

The third area Nordenfelt identifies is the 'clinical context', and he pays special attention to the assumption that the 'essential thing to achieve in the medical pursuit is to solve a problem for the patient and create a bodily and mental state with which he is satisfied' (1993, 22). I will not here attempt to argue for or against this idea. The point is that if participants in the discourse are able to agree about assumptions of this kind, then definitions of the disputed concepts should be consistent with them. Nordenfelt's own definition of health can be used to illustrate the point. Nordenfelt (1993, 22) claims that a person 'is in a state of complete health [...] if and only if, in standard circumstances, he is able to realise his vital goals'. According to Nordenfelt, one reason for accepting this definition is that it matches the intuitive assumption about patient satisfaction. The problem with biostatistical accounts, Nordenfelt holds, is that they cannot match this assumption: '[A] person may be intuitively healthy, without fulfilling the bio statistical criteria for disease and illness' (1993, 22).

The fourth area Nordenfelt mentions is the medical sciences. Nordenfelt holds that it is crucially important that the medical sciences are able to define their domains, that they have an awareness of what aspects of health and disease falls under their scope. But 'how could we understand the science of pathology without a notion of disease? How could we understand the clinical sciences without an idea of their respective spheres?' (1993, 23) The crucial question is again: how should we understand basic health concepts in order to be able to offer plausible characterisations?

In my opinion, Nordenfelt identifies and captures essential aspects of these four areas of discourse very well, and I fully agree that the roles basic health terms have within them constitute reasons for clarifying the corresponding concepts. However, I disagree with Nordenfelt when he claims that the roles constitute reasons for monistic analyses of the concepts. The analytic-synthetic argument implies that one cannot develop general definitions of *the* concept of disease or *the* concept of health that cover an understanding present in all the areas. It is only possible to formulate pluralistic definitions that capture different sets of assumptions about the use of the concepts.

The fundamental difference between this suggestion and Nordenfelt's project is that for Nordenfelt, the contention that a definition captures a common understanding constitutes the justification for applying it within different areas. Finding such a justification is what I have argued cannot be achieved. All one can hope for is that it is possible to formulate different contextual definitions. Such definitions lie in an important sense between pure stipulative definitions and full-blooded conceptual analyses. Their application conditions are not determined by the overall meaning of the concepts, but they aim at the same time to match a specified area.

Of course, it is not given in advance that participants in a particular area of discourse will accept many of the same assumptions about the use of a concept, and if there is comprehensive disagreement then the problem of defining the concept is merely shifted back to determining what the correct background assumptions are. But this pessimism is not justified, at least not *a priori*. Remember that the focus should be on specific areas where one can hope to formulate fundamental aims and challenges without having to focus on the application of the disputed concepts. At any rate, we should seek to explicate such background assumptions before asking the important question whether there is a plausible definition for that area. After all, the assumptions about the correct use of a concept constitute the basis for saying whether a definition is correct.

In sum, what I suggest is that theorists concerned with the nature of disputed health concepts should be more concerned with identifying important areas of medical discourse and then, on the basis of this, elucidating conceptual assumptions within the different areas. It is not unreasonable to hold that such assumptions can be articulated, and if so then there is a normative basis for developing and evaluating definitions. A definition of this kind is not normative in general, but it is not entirely without any normative content as long it yields a correct understanding compared with contextual assumptions about the use of the concept.

Still, if it really turns out to be impossible to find common ground within a context of discourse, then one has not come very far. This problem, one must assume, is most likely to arise in ordinary clinical practice where health professionals encounter a variety of layman beliefs. In this context it takes a great deal of time to uncover underlying special conceptions, and the similarities are often limited (Helman 1984; Lupton 1996). Does the analytic-synthetic argument imply that doctors and patients are seldom able to exchange concepts when they employ terms like 'disease', 'illness' and 'sickness'?

I wish to end by outlining some reasons for not accepting this pessimistic view. Firstly, successful doctor-patient interaction involving the use of a term like 'disease' can sometimes be explained by reference to the fact that the doctor and the patient share an implicit conception of what the word means. Two conceptions that are not explicated in the same way might be more similar than it seems, if future use of the word shows that there are important similarities, or if the doctor or the patient is willing to defer to the other's understanding (Nordby 2003). According to this idea of deference-willingness, a person's willingness to defer to a specific use of a concept is part of his understanding of the concept. If two persons are willing to defer to the same future use, then they can possess the same concept even though they do not explicate the concept in the same way (Burge 1979; Peacocke 1992; Nordby 2003). In order to clarify this important idea of a shared implicit conception of disease, the distinction between 'knowing-how' and 'knowing-that' also becomes relevant. Implicit conceptions can be assimilated to knowing how, to master a technique that cannot be articulated as explicit knowledge but only revealed in a practice (Burge 1986; Peacocke 1998).

Discussing these concepts from philosophy of mind and language in detail would fall outside the focus here. It has been important, however, to make it clear that if the analytic-synthetic argument is correct, then the idea of an implicit conception and the idea of 'knowing-how' should receive comprehensive attention in discussions of doctor-patient communication.

One must at the same time remember that it follows from the analytic-synthetic argument that a doctor is not entitled to insist that his judgement about a grey case is correct. For this to be a justified attitude one needs to show that the doctor's understanding constitutes a normative standard even though it is not part of a common understanding. The analytic-synthetic argument does not imply that it is impossible to articulate an argument of this kind, but I have argued that the prospects look very bleak. After all, our common language is also the language of medical laymen. So why should not patients be entitled to have a non-professional understanding of ordinary language concepts that have a comprehensive history of use outside the medical profession?

I have argued that if definitions of *disease* and other disputed health concepts can be developed, then it is more promising to connect them to special areas of discourse. Furthermore, if a doctor's understanding is not too different from a patient's conceptions then one can always hope, from the perspective of the doctor, that the patient finds his explanations reasonable, defers to them, and therefore acquires the same concepts as the doctor.

References

Albert D A, Munson R and Resnik M D (1988). *Reasoning in medicine: An introduction to clinical inference.* Baltimore: John Hopkins University Press.

Boorse C (1997). 'A rebuttal on health'. In: J M Humber and R F Almeder (eds): *What is Disease?* Totowa, New Jersey: Humana.

Burge T (1979). 'Individualism and the mental'. *Midwest studies in philosophy*, 4, 73–120.

Burge T (1986). 'Intellectual Norms and Foundations of Mind', *The journal of philosophy*, 83, 697–720.

Burge T (1990). 'Frege on sense and linguistic meaning'. In: D. Bell and N. Cooper (eds): *The analytical tradition: Meaning, thought and knowledge.* Oxford: Blackwell.

Campell E J M, Scadding J G and Roberts R S (1979). 'The concept of disease'. *British medical journal,* 2, 757–762.

Davidson D (1984). *Inquires into truth and interpretation.* Oxford: Clarendon Press.

Engelhardt H T (1975). 'The concepts of health and disease'. In: H T Engelhardt and S F Spicker (eds): *Evaluation and explanation in the biomedical sciences.* Dordrecht: Reidel.

Fodor J (1987). *Psychosemantics.* Cambridge, MA: MIT Press.

Freidson E (1987). *Profession of medicine.* Chicago: University of Chicago Press.

Guttenplan S (1996). *A companion to philosophy of mind.* Oxford: Blackwell.

Harman G (1999). *Reasoning, meaning and mind.* Oxford: Oxford University Press.

Helman C (1984). *Culture, health and illness.* Oxford: Butterworth-Heinemann.

Hofmann B (2001). 'Complexity of the concept of disease as shown through rival theoretical frameworks'. *Theoretical medicine and bioethics* 22, 211–36.

Hofmann B (2002). *The technological invention of disease.* Oslo: Oslo University Press.

Honari M and Boleyn T (1999). *Health ecology: Health, culture and human-environment interaction.* New York/London: Routledge.

Juel-Jensen U (1983). *Sygdomsbegreper i praksis.* Munksgaard: Copenhagen.

Kripke S (1982). *Wittgenstein on rules and private language.* Oxford: Blackwell.

Lupton D (1994). *Medicine as culture.* London: SAGE Publications.

Marinker J H (1975). 'Why make people patients?', *Journal of medical ethics* 1, 81–84.

Nettleton S (1995). *The sociology of health and illness.* Cambridge: Polity Press.

Nordby H (2003). 'Doctor-patient-interaction is non-holistic'. *Medicine health care and philosophy,* 6, 145–152.

Nordenfelt L (1987). *On the nature of health*. Dordrecht/Boston/London: Kluwer academic publishers.

Nordenfelt L (1993). 'On the relevance and importance of the notion of disease'. *Theoretical Medicine* 14, 15–26.

Nordenfelt L (2001). *Health, science and ordinary language*. Amsterdam/New York NY: Rodopi.

Nordenfelt L and Twaddle A (1993). 'Disease, illness and sickness: Three central concepts in the theory of health'. *Studies on health and society* Linköping: Linköping University Press.

Peacocke C (1992). *A study of concepts*. Cambridge, MA: MIT Press.

Peacocke C (1998). 'Implicit conceptions, understanding and rationality'. *Philosophical issues* 9, 43–89.

Putnam H (1962). 'The analytic and the synthetic'. In: H. Feigl and G. Maxwell (eds): *Minnesota studies in the philosophy of science*, 3, 358–97.

Putnam H (1975). *Philosophical papers: Vol. 2*. Cambridge: Cambridge University Press.

Resnek L (1987). *The nature of disease*. London: Routledge.

Scadding J G (1967). 'Diagnosis: The Ccinician and the computer'. *Lancet* 2, 877–882.

Quine W V (1953). *From a logical point of view*. Cambridge, MA: Harvard University Press.

Quine W V (1960). *Word and object*. Cambridge, MA: Harvard University press.

Quine W V (1969). *Ontological relativity and other essays*. New York: Colombia University Press.

Quine W V (1985). 'Two dogmas of empiricism'. In: A.P. Martinich (ed): *The philosophy of language*. New York/Oxford: Oxford University Press. Originally published in Quine (1953).

Wittgenstein L (1953). *Philosophical Investigations*. Oxford: Blackwell.

Worrhall J and Worhall J (2001). 'Defining disease: Much ado about nothing?' *Analecta Husserliana* 72, 33–55.

Chapter 5

Wittgenstein's theory of conceptual competence and virtue analyses of ethical dilemmas in nursing practice

Summary The chapter discusses Ludwig Wittgenstein's theory of conceptual competence within the area of nursing ethics. Wittgenstein's analysis shares fundamental assumptions with virtue approaches to ethical dilemmas in caring practice but is at the same time crucially different. The main difference is that while virtue theories have focused on psychological attitudes like compassion and empathy, Wittgenstein focuses on a person's understanding of concepts like *good* and *wrong*. According to Wittgenstein, an ethical competence in nursing is not equivalent to knowledge of moral principles that are understood independently of contexts of application. But Wittgenstein is also opposed to the view that it is contextual knowledge that provides the normative basis for caring. For Wittgenstein, an ethical competence is essentially a 'preconceptual' awareness of how caring concepts apply. According to this analysis, nurses should address ethical dilemmas in patient interaction by focusing on their understanding of ethical concepts in the context of interaction. Case studies are used to clarify this and other practical implications of Wittgenstein's position.

1. Introduction

Ludwig Wittgenstein's *Philosophical Investigations* (1953) is commonly regarded as one of the most important works in modern analytical philosophy. Wittgenstein's analyses of language mastery and concept possession have had an enormous impact on discussions of the nature of human thought and language, not only in the philosophy of mind and other philosophical disciplines, but also more generally within the humanities and social sciences (Flew 1985; Winch 1958; Wulff 1986; Coates 1996).

Ethics is probably the area in which the applied dimension of Wittgenstein's philosophy has received most attention. It is widely agreed that Wittgenstein's analyses pose a fundamental challenge to theories that assume that general moral rules or principles can serve as instruments for ethical justification (Beauchamp 1991; Johnston 1991). Many have held that Wittgenstein convincingly argues that a proper characterization of an ethical competence shows that ethical principles cannot have the normative role that most classical theories have assumed that they have (Barrett 1991; Bennett et al. 1996; McDowell 1998).

The aim of this chapter is to argue that Wittgenstein's theory of conceptual competence constitutes an important supplement to virtue approaches in nursing ethics. According to Wittgenstein, abstract rules cannot capture the competence that underlies nurses' application of ethical concepts like *right* or *wrong* in patient interaction. But Wittgenstein is also opposed to the view that a nurse's competence plays no justificatory role, that it is purely contextual knowledge that provides the basis for evaluative judgments. Wittgenstein, in an important sense, seeks to identify a middle path between ethical particularism and a general rule-based ethics.

This focus on context and skepticism about the normative force of general moral principles can also be found in virtue approaches that have recently become influential in nursing ethics (Reynolds 2000; Burkhardt and Nathaniel 2002; Tschudin 2003). But while virtue approaches have focused on various psychological attitudes like empathy and compassion, Wittgenstein's concern is to analyze a person's ability to apply ethical concepts on the basis of an understanding of the concepts. In the last part of the chapter, case studies are used to clarify the practical implications of Wittgenstein's analysis, paying particular attention to the importance of being contextually aware of how ethical concepts apply in patient encounters.

2. Virtue ethics in nursing

In order to understand Wittgenstein's theory of conceptual competence, it will be helpful to relate his views to virtue approaches to ethical dilemmas in nursing. This section clarifies main assumptions in this tradition. Davis et. al. (1997, 48) define a virtue approach as a position that presupposes that the 'character and integrity of nurses as individual moral agents determine or, at the very least, influence whether ethical problems are identified and how responses are developed to such problems in patient care'. Virtue theorists hold that

> [c]haracter and virtue, often considered to be too subjective, have a place in today's professional health care ethics [...] Descriptions of character and character traits portray a way of being instead of a way of acting [...] The nurse who responds to a difficult patient care situation with respect, patience and attitude of care is described as a 'good' nurse or as a 'good' person (Davis et. al. 1997, 49).

One can extract from this three ideas of what a virtue approach to nursing ethics involves (see also Nortvedt 1998; Burkhardt and Nathaniel 2002; Scott 2003; Haegert 2003). Firstly, virtue theories are concerned not with instruments for ethical justification, but with the question of what it is that that characterizes a 'good' nurse. Secondly, a proper characterization of a 'good' nurse cannot merely focus on observable actions in nurse-patient-interaction. Virtue approaches hold that a virtue such as empathy lies as much in a nurse's attitudes

121

as in her actions (Foot 2002). Thirdly, it is assumed that possession of attitudes essential for caring cannot be reduced to knowledge of moral rules. Virtue theorists have held that it is impossible to specify sets of moral rules such that nurses necessarily possess a given attitude if their actions are guided by those rules.

Attitudes that have received particular attention in virtue analyses include empathy, compassion, discernment and integrity (Davis et. al. 1997; Beauchamp 1991; Tschudin 2003). The various analyses have differed depending on the theoretical frameworks that have been employed and the aims of the analyses. Despite the differences, virtue analyses have shared the assumption that a focus on virtues is needed as an alternative to theories 'characterized by a focus on right decisions and acts based on consideration of more abstract ethical principles' (Davis et. al. 1997, 49). As Scott (2003, 26) observes, this shift of focus has been especially salient in the last few decades:

> [A] number of contributors to the health care ethics literature have, for a number of years now, tried to argue that within the health care and nursing context, a virtue theory approach is needed at least as a supplement to a duty- and principle-based approach.

This recent criticism of rule-based ethics has had two sources. The first is what one can think of as internal arguments that build on ethical problems and challenges that arise within ordinary nursing practice. The internal arguments have claimed, basically, that knowledge of general rules or principles does not constitute a proper action-guiding competence. Rules, it has been maintained, can give the wrong answer (the rule does not recommend the action that is perceived to be correct) or fail to give a clear answer (the rule does not cover the situation in a determinate way).

The type of dilemma that has perhaps received most attention concerns patient autonomy and controversial issues of paternalism. In cases where autonomous patients do not endorse actions proposed by nurses, a utilitarianist can in principle accept paternalism if it is believed that this course of action will have the best consequences (Wulff, Pedersen and Rosenberg 1986). Within utilitarianism, acceptance of paternalism does not necessarily involve a contradiction. A deontologist in the Kantian tradition, on the other hand, will be unable to accept this kind of paternalism. According to a Kantian deontologist, nurses have a fundamental ethical duty to act in accordance with autonomous patient choices.

Virtue approaches claim that the problem of determining whether one should favor ruled-based utilitarianism or a Kantian form of deontology is a pseudo problem, since both positions are principle-based. In order to understand how nurses should solve dilemmas connected to patient autonomy and paternalism, virtue approaches hold that it is more promising to focus on character. A nurse's entitlement to act in a certain way in this and other kinds of nursing dilemmas is not based on knowledge of general rules, but in attitudes that a 'good' nurse possesses.

In addition to the arguments that have arisen from intrinsic aspects of nursing, a second source of arguments for virtue approaches has focused on considerations that are more external to nursing practice. Here the main focus has been the philosophy of Aristotle and theories within the Aristotelian tradition. It is widely held that Aristotle's theory of moral development provides a plausible general description of how humans 'learn to be good' and that it therefore applies within the specific field of nursing ethics as well (Beauchamp 1991; Bennett et al. 1996). Furthermore, virtue theorists have focused on the fact that Aristotle's analysis of human development is not restricted to ethics, but formed within a comprehensive system of how all organisms strive to develop their potential (Burnyeat 1980; Foot 2002).

Even though virtue theories have in this way been based on general philosophical assumptions, there is an important sense in which any virtue approach to ethical dilemmas in nursing practice will focus on the idea of a nursing context. The reason is as follows: as long as virtue theories are hostile to the action-guiding character of abstract rules and principles, they will assume that context-sensitivity plays an essential role in ethical reasoning. Note that if a nurse's ethical competence could provide action-guidance independent of context, then that competence would have the same status as traditional, normative principles. That is, the competence would be abstract and detached from different nursing contexts, much in the same way as principles of deontology or utilitarianism can be described and understood independently of the contexts in which they can be applied. Such a distinction between a general competence and the application of a competence is precisely what virtue theorists have been opposed to. According to virtue approaches, there is no abstract and fundamental core of moral knowledge that can guide nurses in the variety of contexts they encounter. Virtue theories hold that moral insight depends essentially on contextual awareness.

In this general characterization of virtue approaches, the idea of nursing competence should not be understood in a specific, narrow way. Different virtue theories will address the question of how an ethical competence should be analyzed in different ways, depending on the epistemological and metaphysical assumptions they are based on. The important point is that even though all virtue approaches assume that a nurse's competence plays an action-guiding role, this competence is perceived to be essentially incomplete without context (Burnyeat 1980). Moral insight is always derived from reasoning in a particular situation, as experienced and interpreted by the nurse.

How should this process of subjective interpretation more precisely be analyzed? Virtue approaches to ethical dilemmas in nursing practice have not analyzed this relationship between competence and context to any significant extent. The focus has been on character and attitudes conceived of as a competence that 'good' nurses possess, but to think of the 'virtues' detached from contexts of application is to think of them as equivalent to abstract, general norms. A thorough analysis of how the virtues can underlie applications of ethical concepts needs to relate the virtues to actual evaluative judgments. The aim of the next sections is to show that Wittgenstein's theory of conceptual competence sheds important light on this relation.

3. Wittgenstein on conceptual competence

Wittgenstein's theory of language mastery, published in his *Philosophical Investigations* (1953), shares with virtue approaches the idea that our applications of concepts – ethical or non-ethical – are made on the basis of a conceptual competence. Wittgenstein's fundamental philosophical aim is to clarify exactly how this happens, how the use of a concept 'in some unique way is predetermined, anticipated – as only the act of meaning can anticipate reality' (Wittgenstein 1953, 76).

According to Wittgenstein, the problem arises when one seeks to analyze this relation, and he holds that this problem has two aspects. The first phenomenological aspect concerns the 'experience of being guided' (Wittgenstein 1953, 70), how we should conceive of the phenomenological character of the process of applying a concept or a language expression on the basis of our understanding. Wittgenstein argues that this subjective process cannot be thought of as a conscious, mental event. We have no experience of intentionally being instructed by our understanding when we use language. Wittgenstein uses the example of a mental picture of a cube to illustrate this:

> Suppose that a picture comes before your mind when you hear the word 'cube'. In what sense can this picture fit or fail to fit a use of the word 'cube'? – Perhaps you say: 'It's quite simple; – if that picture occurs to me and I point to a triangular prism for instance, and say it is a cube, then this use of the word doesn't fit the picture.' But doesn't it fit? I have purposely so chosen the example that it is quite easy to imagine a method of projection according to which the picture does fit after all (Wittgenstein 1953, 54).

The same point applies if a person claims that a word or a sentence that comes before his mind tells him how an ethical concept applies. A rule formulation cannot in itself tell a person what the correct use of a concept is; it does not contain its own 'method of projection'.

In order to understand Wittgenstein's argument, consider a nurse who is interested in the moral status of a certain course of action in a patient encounter. How can the word 'good' tell the nurse whether or not the concept *good* applies to that action? Suppose the nurse appeals to a rule formulation: 'An action with properties x, y and z is a good action, and the action I consider has these properties'. But the problem is the same. What is the nurse's basis for holding that this sentence implies that the concept *good* applies?

It would not help to refer to the following new sentence: 'When I am disposed to think that an action with properties x, y and z is good, and when I consider an action with properties x, y and x, then the concept *good* applies.' In that case, the nurse has simply introduced another rule formulation, 'one interpretation after another' (Wittgenstein 1953, 81). Once more the nurse has to ask why s/he is justified in interpreting the rule formulation in one specific way, and the problem reemerges. The problem is that in order to make it clear that a rule has normative force – that there is only one particular action that corresponds to the rule – the rule has to be interpreted in a single determinate way. The nurse could attempt to create such an interpretation by introducing a new rule formulation, but then this 'rule for interpreting a rule' also has to be interpreted. We can go on indefinitely trying to ground interpretations of rule formulations in new rule formulations (Wittgenstein 1953; 1956).

The second aspect of the problem of explaining conceptual competence arises when we seek to understand how a concept rule can capture all the different situations in which we are disposed to apply a concept. As a number of Wittgenstein interpreters have noted, this problem is especially striking within ethics (Kripke 1982; McDowell 1998; Johnston 1991; Barrett 1991). How can some limited set of beliefs that a nurse has about the concept *good* make it clear how the concept should be used in all the contexts s/he is disposed to apply to the concept? Many aspects of different situations can constitute a person's basis for applying the concept 'good'. So how can a finite rule in the person's mind cover all these situations? As long as the contexts in which we are disposed to apply the concept differ to such a large extent, it seems impossible to understand how a rule for the application of the concept can capture all the aspects we consider relevant for deciding whether the concept applies (Kripke 1982).

This argument is, in fact, similar to a line of reasoning that many virtue theorists have appealed to in defending their position. Proponents of virtue analyses have often focused on the fact that it seems overwhelmingly difficult to formulate ethical norms that cover possible contexts of applications in ways that are intuitively correct, and they have inferred from this that moral insight is grounded in something other than awareness of correspondence between general norms and properties of particular contexts. The main difference between this argument and Wittgenstein's analysis is that the ethical argument has focused on how actions should be evaluated, not on fundamental issues of understanding and conceptual competence as such.

Wittgenstein's solution to the problem of explaining how our understanding can guide our applications of concepts, represents an attempt to find a middle path between the view that rule-following is a conscious process and the sceptical view that, we merely conform to communal rules. The key to understanding how this is possible, Wittgenstein argues, is to reject a traditional view of how our conceptual competence must guide us in order for action-guidance to occur. According to this traditional view, a rule must be consciously present before a person's mind in order to be normative; it must be possible for the person to derive how he should apply a concept from a rule that has his attention. Wittgenstein argues that if we instead think of rule following as a practice, that the way we apply concepts as 'techniques' or 'customs' determines the content of our understanding, then it is possible to accept that concept applications are rational:

> What this shows is that there is a way of grasping a rule which is not an interpretation, but which is exhibited in what we call 'obeying the rule' and 'going against it' in actual cases. [...] And hence also 'obeying a rule' is a practice. And to think one is obeying a rule is not to obey the rule (Wittgenstein 1953, 81).

Fundamentally, what Wittgenstein means to show is that, conscious rule-guiding is not something we ordinarily look for when we apply concepts: 'While I am being guided, everything is quite simple, I notice nothing special; but afterwards, when I ask myself what it was that happened, it seems to have been something indescribable' (Wittgenstein 1953, 71). According to Wittgenstein, the traditional assumption that the process of being guided by one's own understanding is a conscious process does not correspond to how we ordinarily conceive of language mastery, and it is therefore unjustified.

4. Ethical dilemmas in nursing practice

It is widely acknowledged in the philosophical literature on ethics, that Wittgenstein is sceptical to the use of rules as instruments for justification in ethics. As Beauchamp (1991) observes, Wittgenstein belongs within a philosophical tradition that holds that it is practice and not rule-based theories that should have priority in moral thinking:

> [P]ractice-based philosophers have appealed to major tradi-
> tional philosophers, including Socrates, Hume and Ludwig
> Wittgenstein. These developments are not always hostile to
> traditional moral philosophy, broadly construed, but they are
> essentially hostile to utilitarianism and Kantian ethical theories
> (Beauchamp 1991, 278).

Applied to the area of caring practice, the main consequence of Wittgenstein's analysis is that no description of rules or principles can capture the competence used by a nurse as a basis for applying ethical concepts like *good* and *wrong*. To think that there are rules that guide nurses in this way is to misunderstand the use of ethical concepts, equivalent to 'a certain characteristic misuse of our language that runs through ethical and religious expressions' (Wittgenstein 1956, 9).

According to Wittgenstein, as long as it is impossible to describe an ethical competence as a set of learned rules, the idea that nurses apply ethical concepts on the basis of a conceptual competence has to be understood in an alternative way. There must be something else that explains how a nurse's beliefs, thoughts and experiences can constitute an action-guiding ability in the variety of patient interactions they are involved in. Thus, Wittgenstein is not opposed to all theories that claim that an ethical competence is learned or acquired. His target is the idea that the competence consists of the possession of general rules, and the practical and theoretical problems that arise if one assumes that ethical concepts have a general rule-based meaning.

Wittgenstein's analysis implies that nurses cannot ground the application of ethical concepts in their own conscious minds. There are no aspects of their beliefs, thoughts or experiences that constitute rules that 'contain their own methods of projection', as Wittgenstein's above 'cube'-example illustrated. Knowledge of how an ethical concept applies is essentially constituted by the use of the concept; a nurse needs to have an awareness of how the concept applies before s/he can fully understand how the concept applies. For Wittgenstein, educating nurses ethically is therefore not giving them knowledge of general rules, but showing them how ethical concepts apply: 'If you wanted to bring someone up ethically [...] you would have to teach it to him after having educated him' (Wittgenstein 1980, 81).

The following case involves a familiar dilemma that can be used to illustrate the implications of Wittgenstein's views:

> A nurse working in a hospital attends to an elderly patient who is alone much of the time, with few visits from relatives and friends. The nurse has a busy schedule and is instructed not to spend much time with patients, but it is obvious that this particular patient really appreciates talking to her. The nurse thinks about this dilemma for a while. She then turns her attention to the patient and becomes confident that the right thing to do is to stay with her for a while.

In this situation the nurse meets the patient with a conception of what a good action is. This conception involves mental states such as beliefs and experiences from other situations, if the nurse has encountered similar relevant situations. For the purpose of understanding the implications of Wittgenstein's analysis the precise content of the nurse's conception is not important. Wittgenstein's fundamental point is completely general. He would argue that regardless of the nature of the nurse's conception, it would not constitute a rule with a determinate interpretation. If the nurse consciously interprets beliefs or experiences in a certain way, then s/he has introduced a 'rule for interpreting a rule', but then this further rule also has to be interpreted.

According to Wittgenstein, a nurse who makes such an introspective attempt to ground an application of an ethical concept in beliefs, thoughts or experiences will be unable to determine how s/he should deal with an ethical dilemma. But Wittgenstein argues that the problem that arises is a quasi-problem. If a nurse does not presuppose that a rule can provide action-guidance consciously, the nurse's competence is applied in the following way: the nurse has a particular experience of what a good action is in a given situation, an awareness that makes it clear to the nurse what s/he thinks it is correct to do. This awareness is partly based on beliefs about what a good action is, but it is preconceptual in the sense that it cannot be deduced from the beliefs in any strict logical sense. It is rather the other way around; it is the experience of what the good action is, in the particular situation, that provides the conceptual content of the nurse's beliefs, so that it becomes manifest to the nurse what s/he thinks it is correct to do. The nurse starts to genuinely believe that it is correct to act in a certain way, but that belief is grounded in an initial awareness that it was correct to act in that way.

Ethical dilemmas in nursing practice do not always arise in situations involving a conflict between formal instructions or procedures and interpersonal relations. Wittgenstein's arguments also apply in cases of more classical ethical dilemmas involving a tension between fundamental ethical considerations. Consider the following case:

A patient is scheduled to take a certain medicine at regular intervals. The patient sometimes experiences negative side effects of the medicine, and one day they are particularly acute and uncomfortable. The patient asks a nurse who visits her if she could have a slightly smaller dose than usual. The nurse (and the patient) is well informed about the nature of the patient's condition of illness and the medical importance of the medicine. However, when the nurse weighs this against the patient's negative experiences and her knowledge that one slightly smaller dose will not significantly increase the risk of serious illness, she becomes confident that it is ethically correct to act in accordance with the patient's wishes.

This case represents a type of dilemma that is often experienced in nursing practice. Should paternalistic considerations that focus on consequences sometimes outweigh patient preferences that seem to be reasonably well informed and based on rational reasoning? In this case the nurse thought that the answer was no. In her opinion, the patient's autonomous desire to avoid the side effects outweighed the general medical instructions.

According to Wittgenstein, it is impossible for nurses to find in their own, conscious minds 'instructions' that can tell them what they should do in a situation like this. There are no mental states that can constitute a rule with such an intrinsic property. Obviously, the nurse in the above example engaged in reasoning and made the judgment that it was correct to comply with the patient's wishes, and this was a decision that was more in line with deontological principles than with traditional principles of utilitarianism. But it was not based on some special deontologist rule that could be used to deduce a solution to the dilemma. It was the nurse's experience that the concept *good* applied that provided the content of her belief that it was correct to comply with the patient's wishes. When she formed this belief she had already applied the concept *good*.

Wittgenstein, in effect, recommends a certain order of priority with respect to how we should think about the relation between evaluative judgment and ethical justification. According to the traditional view, deciding what it is correct to do is an epistemological issue (Burnyeat 1980; Beauchamp 1991; Johnston 1991). We first have to determine how a concept should be used, and then use it accordingly. Wittgenstein, however, argues that ethical justification can only be derived from a contextual awareness of how a concept applies. For Wittgenstein, questions of how concepts should be used cannot be separated from questions of understanding and concept possession.

6. Implications

It is important to emphasize that skepticism about the possibility of formulating moral rules is consistent with the possibility of rational dialogue about ethical dilemmas. By clarifying beliefs, thoughts and feelings that explicitly or implicitly underlie evaluative judgments in nursing practice, rational discourse involving communication of such mental states is possible. So Wittgenstein's views do not imply any kind of moral relativism, the extreme view that there is no basis for rational discussion in cases of uncertainty or disagreement.

A second implication of Wittgenstein's views is that they are meant to capture ethical reasoning in general. Normally, nurses merely have an implicit awareness of the practical reasoning that underlies their evaluative judgments, but when challenged to defend or explain their actions they typically refer to beliefs and thoughts as the basis for their actions. Furthermore, when nurses face moral dilemmas, they often consciously reflect on possible solutions if there is time to do so. It is important to emphasize that Wittgenstein's analysis covers both implicit and explicit ethical reasoning. It aims to capture the general relation between an ethical competence and the application of that competence.

The idea that use of ethical concepts can elucidate an ethical competence does not merely apply on the individual level. A central concept in Wittgenstein's philosophy is the idea of a shared 'language game'. For Wittgenstein, persons use a language expression in a shared language game if they use it in a sufficiently similar way. Here the qualification 'sufficiently' is important. Wittgenstein's analysis does not imply that participants in a language game must have an identical understanding, that their understanding 'determines the use causally' in exactly the same way (Wittgenstein 1953, 79). Wittgenstein uses the expression 'family resemblance' to refer to individual 'patterns of use' that are sufficiently similar to belong within a shared language game. For Wittgenstein (1953), belonging to a language game is mastering a 'practice' (81), conforming reasonably well to 'the system of reference by means of which we interpret' (82).

The consequence of this for the status of collective nursing practices is obvious. It follows from Wittgenstein's views that if nurses apply ethical concepts in shared language games, then they also have a shared competence. For Wittgenstein it is therefore possible to understand how nurses have a shared ethical competence by elucidating how ethical concepts are used collectively. Furthermore, insofar as there is widespread agreement that an ethical competence is part of a more general nursing competence, an understanding of the nature of shared ethical practices can tell us something important about the nature of a more general, shared nursing competence.

Obviously, it remains a further empirical question to determine the extent of shared evaluative judgments in nursing practice. The important theoretical point here has been to show that Wittgenstein's views imply that the question of whether or not nurses have the same ethical competence must be settled on the basis of an understanding of how they use ethical concepts, not on the basis of what abstract beliefs and thoughts they have. In this way Wittgenstein's analysis places a substantial theoretical and methodological constraint on how one should pursue empirical investigations related to the idea of an ethical competence in nursing.

Wittgenstein's focus on competence and awareness of how concepts apply can also be found within virtue approaches to ethical dilemmas in nursing practice. As shown above, virtue analyses are sceptical to rule-based theories, and they also focus on attitudes conceived of as part of a competence that underlies 'good' actions. At the same time there are three reasons why Wittgenstein's philosophy is crucially different from virtue approaches.

Firstly, while virtue analyses have focused on a variety of psychological attitudes, Wittgenstein's philosophy can be used to address the more general question of how a nurse's ethical competence can provide action guidance. This is a fundamental question that confronts any analysis of the relation between an action and the attitudes that underlies it. For instance, if one is incapable of explaining how empathy can constitute an action-guiding competence, then one has not given a complete explanation of how empathy can underlie 'good' actions. In this sense Wittgenstein's analysis of a conceptual competence can give us a deeper understanding of the mental processes virtue analyses are concerned with.

Secondly, Wittgenstein focuses directly on thinking. It is standardly assumed that processes of ethical deliberation must involve reasoning as long as they are cognitive processes (Beauchamp 1991; Coates 1996; McDowell 1998; Tchudin 2003). So if a nurse is able to apply concepts intentionally on the basis of beliefs and thoughts, then she is also able to engage in practical reasoning that can constitute the basis for intentional action. Wittgenstein's theory of conceptual competence is therefore more fundamental than explanations of intentional action that presuppose that we are able to engage in practical reasoning, and classical virtue approaches fall within the latter category. That is, virtue theorists have not been concerned about explaining how we are able to think and reason. Their more restricted aim has been to argue that a person (who is assumed to be able to reason and apply concepts intentionally) performs 'good' actions on the basis of psychological attitudes like compassion and empathy.

The fact that Wittgenstein's philosophy focuses on fundamental relations between thought and language has the additional implication that it is relevant for understanding ethical dimensions of nurse-patient communication. Ethical discourse involves language that expresses ethical concepts, and it follows from Wittgenstein's views that ethical agreement is based on contextual experiences of how ethical concepts apply. Consider a nurse and a patient who discuss what the best choice of action is in a given context. According to Wittgenstein, agreement about this must be based on intuitions both parties share, not on the acceptance of a general moral theory. Wittgenstein in effect holds that a nurse and a patient do not understand ethical concepts in the same way unless they agree about how the concepts apply. Agreement is not merely perceived to be the aim and criterion for successful interaction, but the fundamental condition for understanding and communication in the first place.

The third and final fundamental difference between Wittgenstein's theory and virtue approaches is that Wittgenstein's position is developed within a theoretical framework that is different from the Aristotelian philosophical system and other conceptual frameworks that virtue theories have been developed within (Beauchamp 1991; Foot 2002; Scott 2003). This does not mean that Wittgenstein's position and virtue approaches are incommensurable, but it means that specific objections to fundamental assumptions in virtue analyses will often fail to address the premises of Wittgenstein's arguments. Wittgenstein's writings offer an alternative approach for studying phenomena that virtue approaches have focused on, and this approach deserves attention even if one thinks that the arguments for classical virtue theories are implausible. One must also remember that Wittgenstein's arguments have been regarded as convincing by a large number of modern philosophers (Barrett 1991; Beauchamp 1991; Johnston 1991; McDowell 1998). This in itself is a good reason for exploring his philosophy within the field of nursing ethics.

It is not possible to discuss Wittgenstein's views in detail in an chapter of this scope. The more modest aim has been to outline some of the basic ideas in Wittgenstein's position and explain why these ideas constitute an important supplement to virtue approaches. Further research is needed to determine exactly how Wittgenstein's philosophy should be applied within the field of nursing ethics. Hopefully, the analysis presented in this chapter will help to stimulate such research.

References

Barrett C (1991). *Wittgenstein on ethics and religious belief*. Oxford: Blackwell.

Burnyeat M (1980). 'Aristotle on learning to be good'. In: A. Oksenberg Rorty (ed): *Essays on Aristotle's ethics*. Berkeley, LA: University of California Press.

Beauchamp T (1991). *Philosophical ethics*. New York: McGraw-Hill.

Bennett R, Erin C, Harris J and Holm S (1996). Bioethics, genetics and medical ethics. In: N. Bunnin and E. Tsui-James (eds): *The Blackwell companion to philosophy*. Oxford: Blackwell.

Burkhardt M and Nathaniel A (2002). *Ethics and issues in contemporary nursing*. New York: Delman learning.

Coates J (1996). *The claims of common sense: Moore, Wittgenstein, Keynes and the social sciences*. Cambridge: Cambridge University Press.

Davis A, Arosker M, Liaschenko J and Drought T (1997). *Ethical dilemmas and nursing practice*. Stamford, Conn: Appleton and Lange.

Flew A (1985). *Thinking about social thinking: The philosophy of the social sciences*. Oxford: Blackwell.

Foot P (2002). *Virtues and vices and other essays in moral philosophy*. Oxford: Oxford University Press.

Haegert S (2003). 'Whose culture? An attempt at raising a culturally sensitive ethical awareness'. In Tchudin (see separate reference).

Johnston P (1989). *Wittgenstein and moral philosophy*. London/New York: Routledge.

Kripke S (1982). *Wittgenstein on rules and private language*. Oxford: Blackwell.

McDowell J (1998). *Mind, value and reality*. Cambridge: Harvard University Press.

Nortvedt P (1998). 'Sensitive judgment: An inquiry into the foundations of nursing ethics'. *Nursing ethics*, 5, 385–92.

Quine W V (1953). *From a logical point of view*. Harvard: Harvard University Press.

Reynolds W (2000). *The measurement and development of empathy in nursing*. Aldershot: Ashgate.

Scott P A (2003). 'Virtue, nursing and the moral domain of practice'. In Tchudin (see separate reference).

Tchudin V (ed) (2003). *Approaches to ethics: Nursing beyond boundaries*. Edinburgh/London: Butterworth-Heinemann.

Winch P (1958). *The idea of a social science*. London: Routledge.

Wittgenstein L (1953). *Philosophical investigations*. Oxford: Blackwell publishing.

Wittgenstein L (1956). 'A lecture on ethics'. *Philosophical Review*, 74, 3–12.

Wittgenstein L (1980). *Culture and value*. Oxford: Blackwell.

Wulff H, Pedersen, S and Rosenberg, R (1986). *Philosophy of medicine*. Oxford: Blackwell.

Chapter 6

Truth-telling in doctor-patient interaction

Summary The question of whether a doctor tells the truth to a patient can only be answered adequately on the basis of a theory of what it is to be truth-telling. In the light of Henderson's influential argument that it is impossible to tell patients the whole truth, theorists have recently suggested that the idea of a truth-telling doctor should be connected to a doctor's intention to be sincere. This chapter argues that this intentionalist analysis is inadequate. The problem, I argue, is that truth-telling is a *communicative* concept; a doctor has told a patient the truth only if he has communicated the truth. In order to determine whether a doctor has told the truth, it is therefore insufficient to focus on the doctor's subjective intentions. It is necessary to focus on other aspects of the interaction between the doctor and the patient as well, such as the doctor's justification for the belief he intends to communicate, and the patient's understanding of the language the doctor uses. I discuss how a communicative concept of truth-telling should be understood and use case studies to show that the communicative concept has practical implications that are strikingly different from the implications of pure intentionalism.

1. Introduction

Should doctors always be sincere and tell patients the whole truth about their condition of disease or illness? When doctors are confronted with patients or relatives of patients who want to know 'everything', are they sometimes entitled to withhold information? If so, what is an adequate justification for deviating from the principle that we should be sincere and communicate the truth to other persons who want to know the truth?

Questions of truth and sincerity in doctor-patient interaction have received significant attention in bioethics. The aim of the discussions has often been to determine whether there may be exceptional circumstances in which doctors are entitled to violate the fundamental ethical norm that they should communicate the truth to patients (Collins 1927; Young 1998; Kushner and Thomasma 2001; Gillon 2001; Higgs 2006). The main reason for exploring this is obvious. If it is possible to identify such exceptional conditions, then these conditions can play an important, practical role. A doctor who knows that an exceptional condition is met in a given encounter with a patient, also knows that he is justified in not conforming to a moral obligation that we generally do not consider ourselves entitled to violate in normal, everyday discourse (Wulff et al. 2001).[11]

In the last few decades, there has been a growing scepticism about the possibility of formulating many exceptional conditions of this kind (Higgs 1998; Gillon 2001; Kuhse and Singer 2006). This scepticism has its origin in an increasing emphasis on symmetrical relations, patient autonomy, informed consent, and a refutation of the traditional idea that doctors are authoritative experts who always 'know best' (Young 1998; Kuhse and Singer 2006; Nordby 2008). However, even if one is sceptical to the idea that doctors are sometimes entitled to withhold the truth and factual information in clinical encounters, questions of truth and sincerity should not be regarded as unimportant. From

---

[11] It is important to note that the plausibility of the principle that we should aim to communicate the truth does not depend on a specific ethical theory or tradition. The principle will be accepted both by proponents of utilitarianism, deontology and 'virtue' approaches (Mill 1974; Kant 1981; Scheffer 1988; Statman 1997). Correspondingly, the idea of a truthful speaker forms a normative basis in very many theories about communication and understanding (Gadamer 1975; Habermas 1990).

a philosophical point of view, the most important questions remain the same: what is it, fundamentally, for a doctor to be truth-telling? What is the nature of a communicative process in which the truth has been communicated (Field 2001)?

The starting point for many analyses of truth-telling in doctor-patient interaction has been the assumption that if the answers to these questions are unclear, it is difficult to determine whether a doctor has told the truth in a given case. If we know what it is to be truth telling in general, then this knowledge can be used to shed light on particular grey cases, i.e. cases where it is not obvious whether a doctor has been truth-telling or not. In other words, the idea of a truthful doctor should not be understood as a purely abstract concept, a philosophical ideal detached from recognisable aims and judgements we wish to make about ordinary doctor-patient interaction.

Discussions of the need to connect conditions of truth to real problems and dilemmas in doctor-patient interaction have often focused on Henderson's influential argument that 'it is meaningless to speak of telling the truth, the whole truth and nothing but the truth to a patient' (Henderson 1935, 819). According to Henderson, the issues in medical discourse are typically so complex that it is overwhelmingly difficult to tell laypersons the whole truth: in order to be able to fully understand comprehensive and detailed medical information, patients need, more or less, a medical education. Henderson's sceptical conclusion is that it is impossible to achieve this aim in ordinary doctor-patient interaction (Henderson 1935).

Theorists have recently argued that Henderson's sceptical argument is unsound if we define truth as an intentional concept (Bok 1978; Higgs 1998; 2006; Gillon 2001). According to the intentionalist analysis, the relevant moral principle is that we should 'speak truthfully and intend to convey what we understand, or we shall lie' (Higgs 2006, 613). As Bok observes, this principle implies that in order to determine whether the basic moral requirement is met, it is sufficient to know whether a person *intends* to speak the truth: 'The moral question of whether you are lying or not is not settled by establishing the truth or falsity of what you say. In order to settle the question, we must know whether you intend your statement to mislead' (Bok 1978, 6). Intentionalists have argued that this means that the problem of communicating the 'whole truth' to laypeople disappears: as long as a doctor means to state the truth, the basic moral condition related to truth-telling is met (Gillon 2001; Higgs 2006).

The aim of this chapter is to show that even though some of the traditional objections to Henderson's sceptical argument do not apply to the alternative intentionalist analysis, intentionalism is nevertheless inadequate as an analysis of truth-telling. The problem, I argue, can be traced to the importance of making a distinction between three questions. Firstly, what does a doctor think is true? Secondly, what is the truth about the topic of the discourse? Thirdly, how does the patient understand the doctor?

Although the first question can be addressed within the intentionalist framework, I would argue that there are important reasons for holding that an analysis of truth-telling should address the two other questions as well. In the last part of the chapter I focus on these questions and develop a *communicative* analysis of truth-telling. According to this analysis, doctors should not have one, but three fundamental conditions in mind in order to achieve the aim of truth-telling as well as possible. In addition to focusing on (i) their communicative intentions, they need to focus on (ii) their justification for the beliefs they attempt to communicate and (iii) patients' understanding of the language that is used. The chapter concludes that a doctor is justified in holding that he has met the fundamental moral obligation of truth-telling only if he is justified in believing that this overall threefold condition is met.

2. Truth-telling and ethical dilemmas

In their influential *Philosophy of Medicine*, Wulff et al. (2001, 100) describe the following case as a typical ethical dilemma where the question of truth-telling is central:

The patient was a middle-aged man who was believed to have a benign stomach ulcer. He was subjected to a gastric resection (removal of part of the stomach), and the histological examination of the resected part unexpectedly revealed the presence of cancer cells. It could not be excluded that the cancer would recur, but no further treatment was considered possible. After the operation, the surgeon had to decide whether he ought to disclose the true diagnosis to the patient.

The dilemma is obvious. The principle that patients should be informed about all relevant aspects of their medical conditions recommends that the whole truth should be communicated to the patient. But since the probability of there being any more cancerous tissue was so small, would not informing the patient simply cause unnecessary worry? As Wulff et al. (2001, 191) observe, the surgeon might think

> [...] that there is a good chance that the patient had been cured, and in that case disclosing the true diagnosis would only cause a lot of unnecessary worry. If the cancer recurred, it might be necessary to tell the truth later, but why not let the patient live happily as long as possible?

Before discussing in more detail how this and other cases of doctor-patient interaction can involve ethical dilemmas where the question of truth-telling is perceived as central, it is important to clarify some assumptions that the discussion will be based on.

The first of these assumptions concerns the possibility of describing ethical dilemmas that cannot be 'dissolved' by adding further assumptions about the cases. Suppose we assume that the patient in the above case has made it clear, before having surgery, that he wants to know everything about his medical condition. This assumption might obviously influence the way the surgeon conceives of the case. It is more reasonable to choose the option of informing the patient about the cancerous tissue if the patient has emphasised that he wants to know the whole truth.

This point is simply a consequence of the widespread assumption that it is overwhelmingly difficult to formulate general and plausible ethical norms in a straightforward way (Singer 1991; Dancy 2005). Any norm will have the following form: in a given situation, specified by a description D, action A is always the 'correct' action. The classical problem is that D has to be extremely complex in order to avoid intuitive counterexamples to the formulated norm (Singer 1991; Statman 1997; Dancy 2005). The same point applies when one tries to describe ethical dilemmas about truth-telling. Even in a fairly straightforward example of the kind described above, it is necessary to make implicit assumptions about the patient's state of mind and other aspects of the situation to make it clear that the case in reality represents a difficult ethical dilemma.

The reason why this is an important point to make, is that some might think discussions of dilemmas about truth-telling are important only if it is possible to *define* such dilemmas. But then one also has to accept that it is unimportant to discuss ethical dilemmas in general – since all ethical dilemmas are equally difficult to define. This is surely not a plausible consequence. Like discussions of other ethical dilemmas, discussions of dilemmas about truth-telling should be based on the assumption that such dilemmas can be *felt* and experienced from a first-person perspective, in a real-life situation (Kushner and Thomasma 2001).

It is then a further question how these felt dilemmas should be described in language, in order to elucidate why they are dilemmas. Obviously, a description of a dilemma will constitute the starting point for a philosophical discussion of it, but it is not crucial that the description captures all aspects that are considered to be ethically relevant. It is sufficient that the description indicates why the case is felt to be an ethical dilemma.

This point is not always made clear in the literature. Higgs cites the following cases as ethical dilemmas where the question of truth-telling arises:

A single mother wants a certificate to say she is unwell so that she can stay at home to look after her sick child. A colleague is often drunk on duty, and is making mistakes. A husband with a veneral disease wants his wife to be treated without her knowledge. An outraged father wants to know if his teenage daughter has been put on the pill. A mother comes in with a child to have a boil lanced: 'Please tell him it won't hurt' (Higgs 2006, 612).

These brief descriptions give good *indication* of how ethical dilemmas can arise. But Higgs could have made it clearer that a dilemma does not necessarily arise even when the conditions specified in the descriptions are met. Consider the case involving the father who demands to know whether his daughter is using contraception. If we assume that the girl is not fourteen but seventeen years of age, and that she has made it clear that she does not want her parents to know, it is even more reasonable to assume that it is ethically correct to act in accordance with her wishes.[12]

Indeed, if we add this as an assumption, the case might not even be felt to be an ethical dilemma at all. Furthermore, how a case is experienced will depend on the ethical beliefs and moral intuitions of the doctor in question. However, the point is that this and the other cases Higgs described are *typically,* or at least very often, experienced as ethical dilemmas. But this is something Higgs could have made explicit, in order to clarify that he does not have to presuppose that the cases he describes necessarily involve ethical dilemmas.

A second preliminary point I would like to make is that it is important to address ethical dilemmas about truth-telling on the basis of considerations about what it is to be truth-telling in general.

---

[12] There is also the professional confidentiality to consider. In this case it is illegal in Norway to tell the father. However, what is conceived of as ethically correct does not *necessarily* correspond to what procedures, rules or legal principles say. It is, in principle, possible to judge an action to be consistent with the law but nevertheless ethically wrong (it is a fact that persons sometimes make judgements of this kind). It is also possible, from a first person perspective, to judge an action to be inconsistent with the law but ethically acceptable.

When a doctor believes that he has told the truth to a patient, then that belief is formed on the basis of an understanding of what it is for someone to be truth-telling. Similarly, if one thinks that a doctor has not told the truth in a given case, then one has to presuppose that the conditions laid down by a proper analysis of the concept *truth-telling* would not be met. This means that if it is possible to define the concept in a clear and coherent way, then the definition can help doctors in difficult cases. A definition of truth-telling can make it easier to understand what it is to be truth-telling and what it is to not tell the truth (Field 2001).

As an illustration of this point, consider the abovementioned case described by Wulff et al. (2001). Suppose that the doctor said to the patient 'Traces of malignancy have been found in samples from the tissue we removed during the surgery.' Has the doctor *told* the patient the truth? The doctor has obviously uttered the truth. But the patient does not necessarily understand the information that the doctor states in words. The doctor has not conveyed the message he intends to communicate if a word like 'malignancy' is an empty sound for the patient (Nordby 2006a).

Thus, if we can clarify what it really is to be truth-telling, then it is easer to give an answer in this and other grey cases, i.e. cases where it is not obvious what it is to tell the truth or whether a doctor has really communicated the truth. A general analysis of what it is to be truth-telling can form a platform from which doctors and other health personnel can understand what telling the truth in specific cases involves. In this sense, the aim of a conceptual analysis of *truth-telling* is similar to other conceptual analyses of basic health concepts. Concepts like *patient autonomy*, *empathy* and *disease* have all been subject to analyses where the aim has been to clarify what it is to be autonomous, show empathy and have a disease (Nordenfelt 2001; Nordby 2006b).

Any attempt to clarify the application conditions of a concept is in this sense an attempt to move discussions of difficult applications to a more general level. Instead of looking at each particular application, a conceptual analysis seeks to clarify the general content of a concept and then use that clarification to derive answers to questions about the concept's application in disputed grey cases (Nordby 2006b).

Such an analysis of the concept *truth-telling* should not from the outset place any restriction on the metaphysical nature of the concept. The important question is whether it is possible to define necessary and sufficient conditions of any kind for the application of the concept. In the following I will first present a sceptical analysis of *truth-telling*, according to which the concept applies in very few cases of doctor-patient interaction. I will then focus on an objection to the sceptical analysis.

3. Partial truth-telling and the intentionalist alternative

Patients typically encounter health workers as medical laypeople; they do not, normally, have expert medical knowledge of their condition of disease or illness, or of the nature of relevant medical treatments and procedures (Nordby 2008). There are of course exceptions. Doctors become patients, and patients with a medical history sometimes acquire detailed knowledge of the nature of their medical condition. Nevertheless, in typical cases of doctor-patient interaction, the doctor has, especially at the start of the encounter, a great deal more relevant medical knowledge than the patient.

Henderson's influential sceptical analysis of truth-telling in doctor-patient interaction focuses on this expert-layperson dimension of the relationship. Telling laypeople the truth, according to Henderson (1935), is simply impossible:

> It is meaningless to speak of telling the truth, the whole truth and nothing but the truth to a patient [...] because it is [...] a sheer impossibility. Since telling the truth is impossible, there can be no sharp distinction between what is true and what is false (Henderson 1935, 819).

Henderson's point is that within the limits of an ordinary clinical encounter, it is impossible to communicate the understanding the patient needs in order to understand the 'whole truth'. Wulff's above example can be used to illustrate the point. Suppose the doctor aims to tell the patient everything he knows about the possible consequences of the discovery of cancer cells in the tissue that was removed during the surgery. The patient, we can presume, knows something about cancer. He knows that cancer is a very serious disease, he knows that cancer can spread to various parts of the body, and he knows that chemotherapy treatment is typically used in attempts to cure cancer.

However, this is limited knowledge, and for the doctor it would take an enormous amount of time and energy to communicate all possible prognoses and relevant aspects of the patient's medical condition to the patient. According to Henderson, as long as it is impossible to achieve a 'complete understanding' in so many cases, the general aim of doctor-patient interaction should be conceived of in an alternative way. The basic principle should be to do what 'is best for the patient' (Henderson 1935). According to Henderson, it is often not in the patient's best interests to be told the truth, since the patient does not have the competence and capacity to grasp the relevant information.

Henderson's sceptical argument has led to extensive debate. The main reason is obvious. It seems on the one hand clear that Henderson is correct – within the limits of ordinary clinical encounters it is typically overwhelmingly difficult for patients to understand very complex and detailed medical information (Nordby 2008). On the other hand, the argument leaves the issue of informed consent and the aim of patient communication in a vacuum. If communication of factual information is not the basic norm, what is in 'the patient's best interests'?

There are two problems with Henderson's argument. Firstly, it implies that doctors' practices should be revised – the fundamental action-guiding principle should not be to inform and explain to patients the real nature of their medical conditions. Secondly, it seems to legitimate a purely subjective, paternalistic and relativistic perspective on the aim of patient communication. If the aim is to do what is 'best for the patient', then who is to decide what this involves? What if a doctor thinks it is in a patient's best interests to be told a lie? Is it acceptable that each individual doctor should make decisions about this from case to case?

The point is that we need some independent standards that can be used to evaluate what is ethically right and wrong. In Wittgenstein's words, if all use of language that seems correct is correct from a person's perspective, in this case the doctor's, then there can be no such thing as a genuine correct communicative strategy (Wittgenstein 1953; 1969). In fact, doctors can communicate exactly what they want as long as they think it is in the patient's best interests. It follows that the communicative relationship between a doctor and a patient is, and should be, what Habermas calls an asymmetrical 'power' relationship (Habermas 1990); the doctor is an authority who determines how language should be used and understood.

The significance of these problems depends, of course, on how Henderson's assumptions apply in medicine and health care today. One issue concerns the extent of patient education and lay knowledge. When Henderson presented his sceptical argument, the typical patient did not have much medical knowledge. Nowadays patients are often well informed by health personnel about their medical condition, and they use other sources such as the internet to learn more. However, as noted above, there can be no doubt that the layperson-expert analysis still applies. In many cases, patients do not know, and find it difficult to understand, detailed and complex medical information (Nordby 2008). Henderson's argument continues to be relevant in all these cases.

More could be said about the details of Henderson's analysis and the expert-layperson he focuses on. My concern here, however, is a more principled objection to Henderson's argument, recently presented by some theorists (Gillon 2001; Higgs 2006). Instead of holding that truth-telling is equivalent to conveying true and complex medical knowledge to a patient, these theorists have held that the basic moral condition related to truth-telling is that a doctor *intends* to tell the truth. According to this intentionalist objection, the problem with Henderson's sceptical argument is that he demands too much: the less demanding and crucial requirement should be that the doctor intends to be sincere. Thus, commenting on Henderson, Higgs writes:

> But we must not allow ourselves to be confused, as Henderson was, and as so many others have been, by a failure to distinguish between truth, the abstract concept, of which we shall always have an imperfect grasp, and telling the truth, where the intention is all important. Whether or not we can ever fully grasp or express the whole picture, whether we know ultimately what the truth really is, we must speak truthfully, and intend to convey what we understand, or we shall lie (Higgs 2006, 613).

A similar strategy has been suggested by Gillon (2001, 511):

> [T]he crucial moral issue concerns the doctor's intentions – in particular, does he intend to discover what the patient would wish to know, and does he intend to try to meet such wishes when they concern the transmission of information that the doctor believes to be both true and likely to distress the patient, or does he intend to deceive the patient?

Both Higgs and Gillon link their arguments to Sissela Bok's (1978) more general intentionalist analysis of truth and make it clear that they think her arguments are compelling. Ultimately, in order to determine whether it is correct for the intentionalist to rest his case on Bok's theory, it is therefore necessary to focus on her arguments.

Independently of these arguments there is, however, a further question we should address. Does the intentionalist analysis constitute a proper framework for analysing truth-telling at all? It seems clear that the intentionalist is correct in holding that a basic moral obligation is met if a person acts on the basis of attitudes like sincerity and honesty (Singer 1991; Statman 1997). Sincerity is a concept that has been analysed in different ways, but it is widely assumed that sincerity is a basic virtue that it is important for health personnel to possess (Enelow et al. 1996). However, how does it relate to truth-telling?

Unlike the applied intentionalist analysis of truth-telling in doctor-patient interaction, Bok's theory is not a theory of truth-telling. Like philosophers such as Løgstrup (1997), Bok's idea is that being sincere is the most basic, moral precondition for all successful human communication and understanding. Of course, the fact that Bok's intention is not to analyse truth-telling does not necessarily mean that her theory is irrelevant for this purpose. But there is at least a possibility here. An analysis of the significance of sincerity is not *necessarily* an analysis of what it is to *tell* the truth. The theorists who have argued for intentionalism have assumed that an analysis of sincerity captures truth-telling as well, but it is far from clear that this is correct.

4. The problem with intentionalism

Suppose that a doctor sincerely believes that a variety of illnesses and diseases can be cured by alternative medicine. He has a patient with an illness of a relevant kind, and he tells the patient that there is a very good chance that his condition will improve if he tries a certain alternative cure. The patient listens and forms the belief that the doctor has told him the truth. But has the doctor told the patient the truth when he sincerely says that there is a good chance that his condition will improve?

Or imagine a doctor in post-operative dialogue with a patient who has undergone surgery for a complex medical condition. The doctor tries to adjust his communication to the patient's perspective, but sometimes he does not succeed. From the patient's point of view, the doctor gives complex information and uses a special language that the patient does not understand very well. He hears the language the doctor is using, but he is weak, and it is difficult for him to understand and systematise all the detailed information he is given.

When the doctor leaves he has many unanswered questions, and he has not understood very much of what the doctor said.

I do not mean that these cases are representative for how doctors typically communicate with patients. The point is that they illustrate an important point about truth-telling. Notice that in both cases the doctor has, apparently, met the intentional condition for truth-telling. The reason is that the doctor genuinely believes what he says, and his intention is to tell the patient the truth. But has the doctor *told* the truth? The problem is that intentionalism does not capture two crucial aspects of truth-telling. First, we typically think there is an objective basis for determining whether someone who thinks he is truth-telling really is truth-telling (Dancy 1991; Field 2001). Second, even when a doctor knows the truth and states the truth in language, it is *communication* that is crucial.

The intentionalist might reply that we should distinguish between sincerity, the abstract concept of truth and communication of truth, and that his focus is only on the first of these. But in that case it seems that his analysis is not an analysis of truth-*telling*. Furthermore, we need a concept of truth-telling. We should grant the intentionalist that it is of fundamental importance that doctors should be sincere, that they should know what it is to be sincere, and that they should be able to state the truth when they know what the truth is. It is important to analyse the concept of sincerity within bioethics, and it is important that doctors should meet plausible ethical conditions of sincerity in real-life encounters with patients. But none of this is equivalent to actually fulfilling the further moral obligation of telling the truth. Telling the truth to someone is not the same as merely uttering in words what one sincerely thinks is true. As illustrated above, what a doctor thinks is true can sometimes be false.

If the intentionalist maintains that this is not how he understands the concept *truth-telling*, that the concept only applies to a person's subjective communicative intentions, then we should respond that his use of the concept does not correspond to its everyday meaning. He takes the concept 'on holiday' as the philosopher Wittgenstein (1953) would say. In its ordinary meaning, telling the truth is an interpersonal and communicative concept. It refers to something speakers have to be able to do in order to convey something to an audience in a communicative process.

Some might object that even if it is correct that truth is a relational concept, we have not solved the basic problem of avoiding Henderson's paternalistic conclusion that doctors should do what they think is 'best for the patient' unless we find a convincing objection to his argument that it is impossible to communicate the whole truth. There are two challenges here. First, it is often unclear what the truth of the matter of discourse is. Is it true to tell patients with whip-lash or chronic low back pain who want to know whether they have a disease, that they have a disease? There are many basic health concepts that do not have clear or defined application conditions (Nordenfelt 2001; Nordby 2006b). Or consider cases where it is difficult to establish a precise diagnosis or prognosis related to a state of ill-health. How long is it reasonable to assume that a patient with terminal cancer can expect to live? What is the prognosis for a patient with many complex and acute injuries due to a serious accident? Many of the questions that patients or relatives of patients want to know the answers to do not have straightforward, factual answers.

Second, a patient will necessarily interpret what a doctor says on the basis of an idiosyncratic horizon that is shaped by a specific social and cultural context (Nettleton 1995). So how can a doctor be confident that he has communicated the truth to a patient as he – the speaker – understands the truth? How can he know that the patient does not interpret his verbal or non-verbal actions in a way that is strikingly different from how he intends them to be understood?

Both of these communicative challenges have received extensive attention in philosophy of medicine and analyses of doctor-patient interaction, and it is often far from clear how the challenges should be met (Nordby 2006a). So perhaps it is better to stick to intentionalism as a more modest analysis? After all, it is easier for doctors to know, purely on the basis of direct knowledge of their own intentions, that they intend to be sincere. As philosophers have emphasised, we normally have privileged first-person access to our own communicative intentions (Davidson 1987; Burge 1996).

This objection, however, is unconvincing. It is not correct that it is impossible to elucidate important aspects of a communicative process involving the communication of truth in patient interaction. In fact, in order to make reasonable judgements about truth-telling in communication, it is normally sufficient to focus on three aspects of the dialogue with the patient.

The first is the doctor's justification for believing that a message he intends to communicate is true. As the above example involving alternative medicine illustrates, believing that something is true is not necessarily the same as knowing that it is true. According to the classical analysis of knowledge, in order to know that a belief is true we need to have a sufficiently good reason for thinking that it is true (Dancy 1991). Obviously, a doctor might be uncertain about the prognosis for a patient, or even doubt that medical examinations have uncovered the truth about the patient's condition. But this is compatible with holding that knowledge and communication of the truth should be the ideal. It is still possible to accept that doctors should aim to communicate beliefs that are as well justified as possible.

The second aspect of doctor-patient interaction that is crucial for understanding what communication of truth involves concerns the doctor's use of language. In the above example involving post-operative dialogue, the doctor knew the truth, but he failed to express it in a way that was comprehensible to the patient. More generally, a doctor might state the truth, and know that he states the truth, but fail to express his true belief in a language that the patient understands in a sufficiently similar way. It is important to remember that a patient's understanding of the language that a doctor uses is shaped by the patient's social context, and this understanding might be very different from the doctor's understanding. Often patients have a very weak understanding of medical vocabulary, and sometimes their understanding is partially incorrect (Nordby 2008).

The third crucial aspect of communication of truth concerns patients' predispositions to form associations about messages that are directly expressed in language. Even when a doctor and a patient understand the language that is used in a sufficiently similar way, even when they have a common language and both understand what is strictly speaking *said*, the patient may nevertheless interpret this message in a way that is very different from the way the doctor intends it to be understood. Here is a typical case:

> A doctor tells a patient in hospital 'Your condition has really improved'. The patient hears the doctor, and he understands the words the doctor is using. Consequently, the patient understands that the doctor intends to communicate the belief that his condition has improved. The patient thinks to himself that this must mean that he will be able to leave the hospital very soon, and he starts to make practical preparations for doing so. It turns out, however, that this was not how the doctor intended his message to be interpreted. The doctor associated the statement that the patient's condition had improved with a form of improvement that did not indicate that the patient should be discharged very soon. But the patient gets frustrated and tells relatives that the doctor gave him false expectations.

The problem here is that the beliefs the patient associates with the statement that is literally expressed in language are very different from the beliefs the doctor associates with the statement. The patient reads more into the language that the doctor is using than what is actually *said*. Now making such rich interpretations is a perfectly natural phenomenon. If we had to utter all the beliefs we wanted to communicate in everyday communication, it would be overwhelmingly difficult to express all our beliefs. We therefore try to be as economical as possible in our communication with others; we try to use as few sentences as possible to communicate everything we want to communicate (Sperber and Wilson 1991). In this sense verbal language is the tip of the iceberg in human communication (Nordby 2008). The problem arises when an audience forms incorrect beliefs about the part of the communicative iceberg that is beneath the surface, when the beliefs that are ascribed to a speaker are very different from the beliefs that the speaker actually has.

This phenomenon is relevant in explanations of what it is for a doctor to be truth-telling. Consider the following case:

> A young girl has serious kidney failure and needs a donor. The child's mother does not have a kidney that matches her daughter's, but she makes it clear that she would have been willing to donate a kidney. The child's father has a kidney that matches, but he tells the doctors that he does not want to be a donor. He also tells the doctors 'Please do not tell my wife that I do not want to donate my kidney'. The mother obviously wants to know about her husband, and the doctors could have appealed to professional confidentiality and not said anything about the father's unwillingness. However, in this case the doctors choose to do the following. They inform the mother that her husband is unsuitable. They do not, however, tell her that the reasons are psychological and not physiological. The mother thinks that the reasons are physiological, and the doctors understand that it is likely that the mother forms this association. But they have told the truth in the sense that they have *stated* something that is true: it is a fact that a person is not suitable as a donor if the person is unwilling. It is just that the mother forms associations about the statement 'Your husband is unsuitable' that are false. So the doctors have not really *communicated* the whole truth.

This is a delicate case, because the doctors have not lied, and in this sense it is not obviously wrong to act as the doctors do from an ethical and communicative point of view. The doctors nevertheless know, or they are at least likely to suspect, that the mother forms associations that are false. This simply shows how complex the issue of truth-telling is, and that doctors need to be aware of patients' wider interpretations in order to understand whether they have communicated the 'whole truth' by their use of language. It is not sufficient to make a statement that is true. It is also necessary to focus more holistically on the way patients understand the meaning of the language that is used, and how they are disposed to form further beliefs about the written or spoken messages that are directly expressed in language.

5. Improving communication

I have argued that the basic problem with intentionalism is that truth-telling is a communicative concept. Note that this criticism cannot undermine Henderson's original argument which intentionalism was developed as a response to. Remember that Henderson's focus was on communication and the patient all the time – his argument was that patients do not have the capacity to grasp the whole truth.

The crucial difference between Henderson's argument and the alternative communicative analysis I have outlined, is that Henderson fails to acknowledge that there are many things doctors can do to improve communication of truth. In short, Henderson went too quickly from the idea that communication of the whole truth can be very challenging, to the far more extreme view that the aim of telling the truth should be rejected altogether.

We should grant Henderson that communicating the whole truth to a patient can be very challenging. The challenges that arise are the same as in all linguistic expert-layperson relations (Putnam 1981; Nordby 2008). However, unlike Henderson's sceptical argument, the communicative analysis can be used to give us a better understanding of why it is difficult to communicate the truth. Furthermore, and more important, the analysis has implications for how communication of truth should be improved. The reason is that the analysis is not sceptical of the aim of truth-telling *in principle*. The (positive) aim should be to ensure that conditions for truth-telling are met as well as possible, within the real-life limits of clinical encounters.

Corresponding to the three aspects of communication of truth discussed above, I suggest that there are three practical communication conditions which doctors should have in mind in order to secure communication of truth as well as possible. The first is to investigate their own basis for accepting beliefs they intend to communicate. This, in fact, falls under the general norm that our beliefs should be justified. In a general sense, of course, we always think our beliefs are justified. If we think there is no good reason whatsoever for having a belief, then we will not have that belief. Thus, we do not normally attempt to communicate our beliefs to other persons unless we think there are good reasons for having these beliefs. But this is not the concept of justification that is crucial in doctor-patient interaction. It is not sufficient that a doctor has a subjective experience of being entitled to have a belief. The relevant concept is more narrow. A doctor's justification should be related to *standards of justification* (Dancy 1991; Chalmers 2000). It is the way a belief is justified that is crucial. The relevant concepts are *objective reasons* and *empirical methods* of justification, as these concepts typically are understood within the medical profession (Freidson 1988).

Obviously, these scientific concepts are not always applicable. There are many topics in doctor-patient discourse that cannot, or should not, be discussed by using a scientific vocabulary or within a scientific context (Nordenfelt 2001). However, this not the crucial point. The point is that if a medical belief should be subject to scientific scrutiny, and if a doctor fails to acknowledge this, then a professional ethical norm has been violated. In the above example involving the doctor who believes in alternative treatment, it is clear that ordinary scientific methods do not establish the validity of alternative medicine. This is something doctors should acknowledge. A doctor might have a subjective belief in the effect of alternative medicine, but this is not sufficient. Medical doctors represent the medical profession, and this is how patients normally think of them. Patients have the right to know that according to widespread professional opinion, medicaments from alternative medicine have no documented effect.

The second practical communication condition doctors should have in mind when attempting to communicate the truth as well as possible, concerns the necessity of having a shared language with the patient. It is easy for doctors to forget that medical terms are sometimes entirely unfamiliar to patients with no medical background.

Doctors do not, generally, use Latin terms without explaining what they mean. They are aware that patients do not understand such terms very well. It is easier for doctors and other health personnel to forget that patients tend to have a weak or very idiosyncratic understanding of subjective expressions like 'pain', 'dizzy', 'hurt' and 'ill' that refer to personal experiences, and common medical terms like 'heart attack', 'inflammation' and 'blood pressure' that have precise definitions within the medical profession. The way patients understand these terms are to a large extent determined by their social and cultural context, and doctors have typically limited knowledge of this context (Nordby 2006a).

The main reason why the use of common medical terms often leads to poor communication is that health personnel who use and hear them a lot easily think 'everyone' knows what they mean (Nordby 2008). Patients with a weak understanding often sense this attitude, and they therefore hesitate to ask what the terms mean. Doctors will typically think they have communicated a substantial meaning by a term like 'blood pressure', but for many patients this is not a word that is particularly informative. Furthermore, patients often have a partially incorrect and sometimes too negative understanding of common health terms. As Gillon (2001, 508) observes,

> [...] even common words such as 'cancer' are likely to be radically misunderstood by patients unless they have had a medical training. The wide range of conditions and prognoses and all other technical nuances implied by the word are probably not taken into consideration and are often replaced by a single dark understanding that cancer is simply another word for a peculiarly horrible death.

It is important for doctors to have an awareness of how patients form negative associations about medical terms. When patients misunderstand medical vocabulary or have a very weak understanding, there can be no platform of a shared language that the communication is based upon.

It is also important to remember that in encounters with health workers, patients who experience negative emotions like pain, shock or anxiety use much of their mental energy to cope with their situation and be present mentally. Their capacity for understanding complex medical terminology is therefore limited. Furthermore, many patients have a reduced capacity for systematising information and rational reasoning due to an experience of illness or injury. An explanation that is straightforward for a doctor might be overwhelmingly difficult to grasp for a patient who has a severe negative first-person experience of illness. Three concepts are essential for doctors when trying to ensure communication. Towards the end of a conversation it is important to *clarify* essential information, provide a *summary* of the most important facts and *control* that the patient has understood the most important information.

I have so far focused on the importance of communicating justified beliefs and the need of having a shared language. The third practical communication condition doctors should have in mind when trying to secure communication of truth, concerns the associations patients form about written or spoken messages. In the example above involving the question of kidney donation it was evident that if the doctors had wanted to improve communication with the mother, they should have clarified the further associations they had. The case is special because it illustrates that it is not, necessarily, always correct to improve communication. However, for the present argumentative purposes it is sufficient to note that the case illustrates the following important point about associative misinterpretation: if there is reason to believe that a patient forms associations that are radically different from a doctor's perspective, and if the doctor wants to improve communication, then the doctor should clarify his own perspective so that it is reasonable to assume that it is this perspective that ends up in the patient's consciousness (Nordby 2006a). This is a practical, action-guiding principle doctors should have in mind when trying to understand whether they have communicated the whole truth.

Obviously, the application of this principle depends on the context of interaction. If a doctor's interpretation of a message corresponds to a widespread social and linguistic norm for how the message should be understood, then it is *prima facie* likely that the patient's associations will not be very different. But if it is not clear that there is such a norm, or if it is reasonable to think that the patient's interpretation is not the common 'ordinary' interpretation, then it is much more important to detect, clarify and possibly adjust the patient's interpretation.

Thus, in the above case involving the sentence 'Your condition has really improved', it is not clear that there exists a common norm of interpretation that supports the patient's interpretation. After all, there is no standard interpretation of a statement like 'Your condition has really improved' that implies that a patient who hears it, in the kind of context in which it was uttered, is entitled to think that he can be discharged from the hospital very soon. So it is not clear that the doctor is to blame for the poor communication in this case.

However, in the other case it is clear that a common social norm of interpretation was violated. When the doctors told the wife that her husband was unsuitable, they should have known that she would think that her husband was unsuitable physiologically and not psychologically. After all, thinking that the reason is physiological is the normal way of interpreting the statement 'Your husband is unsuitable as a donor'. With respect to the wife's misunderstanding, the doctors are therefore to blame.

Of course, much more could be said about practical communication skills and communication conditions. This would, however, fall outside the scope of this chapter. The point has been to show that there are many communicative strategies doctors can choose in order to ensure communication of truth as realistically as possible. The problem arises if we think that the fact that it is difficult to tell laypersons the whole truth implies the far more extreme idea that the aim of truth-telling should be rejected altogether. In many cases it is possible to approximate the aim of telling the truth reasonably well. Doctors can build a fairly good bridge between their own horizons and the patient's perspective by examining their own reasons for uttering a sentence, and by meeting communication conditions like the need to have a shared language.

6. Conclusion

Philosophical attempts to clarify ethical dilemmas involving the question of truth-telling have important practical implications. Philosophical analyses can help doctors to interpret real-life cases where the dilemmas are experienced in patient interaction. In this way an analysis of the concept *truth-telling* can make it easier for doctors to understand what truth-telling is, and what they should do in order to communicate what is true and not false.

If the meaning of the concept of truth-telling was clear, it would not be important to make a conceptual analysis of its meaning. However, the fact that theorists have focused on truth-telling in strikingly different ways shows that the concept does not have a clear pretheoretical meaning. The different perspectives concern the nature and extension of the concept. I have shown that while Henderson's analysis focuses on the expert-layperson dimension of doctor-patient interaction, proponents of intentionalism have argued that it is sufficient that a doctor intends to tell the truth.

I have argued that the arguments for intentionalism are unconvincing. The reason is that truth is a communicative concept. Aiming to tell the truth is not the same as communicating the truth. In fact, stating what is in reality the truth, is not the same as communicating the truth to the patient. I have argued that in order to ensure communication of the truth as well as possible, doctors should have three conditions in mind: they need to have more than a subjective justification for beliefs they intend to communicate, they need to use a language that patients understand, and they need to make sure that patients do not form associations that are radically different from their own associations.

In the last part of the chapter I compared this perspective with Henderson's sceptical argument that the aim of telling the truth should be rejected altogether. Granted, Henderson's focus was on the possibility of communication, but I have argued that his pessimistic and paternalistic conclusion that the general aim should be to do 'what is best for the patient' should be rejected. According to the alternative communicative analysis I have outlined, telling the truth should be the fundamental aim; there is much doctors can do in order to be as truthful as realistically possible. Obviously, there can be many real-life obstacles – among them great differences in knowledge, impaired patient autonomy and limited time to explain – but in very many cases it is possible for doctors to communicate the truth, or at least approximate this aim, by meeting communication conditions and using practical communication skills.

References

Bok S (1978). *Lying: Moral choices in public and private life*. Hassocks: Harvester Press.

Burge T (1996). 'Our entitlement to self-knowledge'. *Proceedings of the Aristotelian Society*, 96.

Chalmers A (2000). *What is this thing called science?* Buckingham: Open University Press.

Collins J (1927). 'Should doctors tell the truth?' *Harper's monthly magazine*, 155.

Dancy J (1991). *A companion to epistemology*. Oxford: Blackwell.

Dancy J (2005). *Ethics without principles*. Oxford: Oxford University Press.

Davidson D (1987). 'Knowing one's own mind'. *Proceedings and addresses of the American Philosophical Association, 2*.

Enelow A, Forde D and Brummel-Smith K (1996). *Interviewing and patient care*. Oxford: Oxford University Press.

Field H (2001). *Truth and the absence of fact*. Oxford: Clarendon Press.

Freidson E (1988). *Profession of medicine*. Chicago: Chicago University Press.

Gadamer H G (1975). *Truth and method*. London/New York: Continuum.

Gillon R (2001). 'Telling the truth, confidentiality, consent, and respect for autonomy.' In: J Harris (ed): *Bioethics*. Oxford: Oxford University Press.

Habermas J (1990). *Moral consciousness and communicative action.* Cambridge: Polity Press.

Henderson L (1935). 'Physician and patient as a social system'. *New England journal of medicine.*

Higgs R (1998). 'Truth-telling'. In: H Kuhse and P Singer (eds): *A companion to bioethics.* Oxford: Blackwell.

Higgs R (2006). 'On telling patients the truth'. In: H Kuhse and P Singer (eds): *Bioethics: An anthology.* Oxford: Blackwell.

Kant I (1981). *Grounding for the metaphysics of morals* (translated by J Ellington). Indianapolis: Hackett Publishing Company.

Kuhse H and Singer P (2006). *Bioethics: An anthology.* Oxford: Blackwell.

Kushner T and Thomasma D (2001). *Ward ethics: Dilemmas for medical students and doctors in training.* Cambridge: Cambridge University Press.

Løgstrup K E (1997). *The ethical demand.* Notre Dame and London: Notre Dame Press.

Mill J S (1974). *On liberty.* London: Penguin Books.

Nettleton S (1995). *The sociology of health and illness.* Cambridge: Polity Press.

Nordby H (2006a). 'Interactive and face-to-face communication'. *Seminar.net,* 3.

Nordby H (2006b). 'The analytic-synthetic distinction and conceptual analyses of basic health concepts'. *Medicine, health care and philosophy,* 2.

Nordby H (2008). 'Medical explanations and lay conceptions of disease and illness'. *Theoretical Medicine and Bioethics,* 6.

Nordenfelt L (2001). *Health, science and ordinary language.* Amsterdam/New York: Rodopi.

Putnam H (1981). *Reason, truth and history.* Cambridge: Cambridge University press.

Scheffer S (1988). *Consequentialism and its critics.* Oxford: Oxford University Press.

Singer P (1991). *Philosophical ethics.* New York: McGraw-Hill.

Sperber D and Wilson D (1991). 'Loose talk'. In: S Davis (ed): *Pragmatics: A reader.* Oxford: Oxford University Press.

Statman D (1997). *Virtue ethics: A critical reader.* Edinburgh: Edinburgh University Press.

Wulff H, Pedersen S and Rosenberg S (2001). *Medicinsk filosofi*. København: Munksgaard.

Wittgenstein L (1953). *Philosophical investigations*. Oxford: Blackwell.

Wittgenstein L (1969). *On certainty*. Oxford: Blackwell

Young R (1998). 'Informed consent and patient autonomy'. In: H Kuhse and P Singer (eds): *A companion to bioethics*. Oxford: Blackwell.

Chapter 7

The ethical dimension of paramedic-patient interaction

Summary In their daily encounters with patients paramedics face the distinction between an ethics that focuses on patients' right to choose the actions they endorse (Kantian deontology) and an ethics that focuses on the consequences of actions (utilitarianism). The dilemma a paramedic sometimes faces can be stated like this: should I act in accordance with the patient's wishes, or should I do what I think has the best consequences for the patient's health? The aim of this chapter is to argue that this dilemma has a practical ethical solution in an important range of cases. These cases have one of two properties: (1) the patient is not able to reason rationally and make free, independent choices in the encounter with the paramedics, or (2) the patient will later realize that the course of action suggested by the paramedics corresponded to his best, overall interests. In these cases paternalism – acting contrary to the patient's expressed preferences – is justified both according to utilitarianism and Kantian deontology. The discussion emphasizes the practical usefulness of this strategy: paramedics typically have to act quickly and efficiently, but in many patient encounters it is reasonable to assume that (1) or (2) is met.

1. Background

As part of a higher education program for paramedics in Norway, I delivered a course on ethics in the spring 2003. On the basis of the discussions among the students and the essays they wrote, it was evident that one of the themes they were most interested in was the classical distinction between utilitarianism and Kantian deontology (Mill 1978; Kant 1996). For the purposes here these two positions can be defined as follows: utilitarianism is the view that one should act in ways that has the best consequences for the person the action is directed towards. Within bioethics, 'patient-utilitarianism' is a well-known version of this general idea (Wulff et al. 1990).

Kantian deontology, on the other hand, is the view that one should act in accordance with the expressed preferences of the person the action is directed towards, if the person has his autonomy intact (Harman 1977; Clarke and Linzey 1996). For a patient to have his 'autonomy intact', I will assume here, is to have a capacity to reason rationally and to make free, independent choices on the basis a proper understanding of his own condition and the possible consequences of various relevant actions (Harman 1997; Sanders 2001). This understanding will be sufficiently precise for the arguments and analyses below.

The reason the students found this difference between utilitarianism and deontology important was that the distinction captured tensions they felt in their daily interactions with patients. Sometimes they felt it wrong to act in accordance with a patient's wishes. In such cases the students thought that other actions than the action the patient endorsed clearly had the best consequences for the patient's health. However, in other cases they thought it was wrong to choose the action they thought had the best consequences for the patient. In such cases the patient clearly desired an alternative action, and the consequences of this alternative action were not conceived to be dramatically more negative than the consequences of the action that had the best consequences for the patient from the perspectives of the paramedics.

The aim of this chapter is to argue that for paramedics, this tension between utilitarianism and deontology can be resolved in an important range of cases. The above definition of deontology requires that in order for it to be ethically correct to accept a patient's wishes, the patient must the autonomous (Harman 1977). But in many emergency situations it is far from clear that the patient is autonomous and capable of free, rational reasoning. I will argue that in such cases the difference between utilitarianism and deontology makes no practical difference in paramedic-patient-encounters: both positions imply that it is ethically correct to choose the action that has the best consequences for the patient's health.

2. Is this a useful discussion for paramedics?

Before I proceed to discuss utilitarianism and deontology in connection with paramedic-patient-interaction in more detail, an objection should be addressed. This objection says that ethical theory and ethical reflection are useless as efficient 'conceptual tools' for paramedics since their actions have to be based on quick, efficient decisions. There is no time, according to this sceptical objection, for a paramedic to engage in philosophical reflection on ethics when he is faced with a patient who needs urgent treatment and transport.

The latter claim is correct (Sanders 2001). But it does not imply that paramedics cannot act efficiently on the basis of a well-founded competence in ethics. Such a competence can result in a better capacity to see aspects of situations that are relevant for making an adequate ethical decision quickly and in an efficient way. Consider the following case (McKenna and Sanders 2001):

Case 1 Your patient has a severe headache, is vomiting, and has a numb right hand. Blood pressure is 220/140 mm Hg. The patient seems to be confused and agitated. Despite your detailed explanations, the patient is refusing treatment and transport.

One important aspect of this situation is that the patient seems confused. Another is that acceptance of the patient's wishes can have very serious consequences for him. It will be argued below that knowledge of these aspects, together with a better understanding of the difference between utilitarianism and deontology, justify the paramedic in holding that it is ethically correct to act contrary to the patient's expressed wishes.

Notice that I say 'ethically correct'. The reason I do this is to stay clear of another objection. This objection, which I have heard stated, says that ethics has no practical use for paramedics, since 'It is the law that tells us what do to anyway'. According to this sceptical objection, ethical reflection is not an important part of the actual reasoning that underlies paramedics' actions in real life situations.

There are several things to be said about this objection. First, it is incorrect that the law always gives straightforward directions for how one should act. The written laws are made up of rules, these rules have to be contextually interpreted, and in such interpretation there is room for uncertainty. In fact, sometimes there is an apparent conflict between different aspects of the written law, and in such cases it especially difficult to use law formulations as straightforward action-guiding resources.

Second, the law is meant to be ethically correct. Justifying an ethical choice by reference to the law is therefore to go in circle unless it is assumed that the law is ethically sound. Taking the further step of thinking about the ethical dimension of the law requires further ethical reflection.

Third, the law says something about the duties of paramedics, but also something about patients' rights (Befring and Ohnstad 2001; Ohnstad 2002). A paramedic might find it ethically correct to do something that is in conflict with actions patients have a legal right to choose.

Fourth, perhaps the most important response to the sceptical objection is that we should make a principled distinction between what is ethically correct and what is legally correct. The obvious reason is that we should not rule out the possibility that the law fails to cover a situation in an ethically acceptable way. Failure of the law to cover different contexts in a way that is ethically acceptable should, in the end, result in changes to the law. Furthermore, it is paramedics working in the first-line services who are in the best position to observe the implications of the relevant laws relating to emergency treatment and transport of patients. One important consequence of this is that paramedics should inform managers, responsible physicians or other relevant persons about experienced inconsistencies between the law and what is ethically correct, so that there can be a more general consciousness about controversial cases.

I have elaborated somewhat on the practical relevance of ethical reflection for paramedics. The main reason is that I have met quite a few health workers who have expressed skepticism about the usefulness of ethical theory in health services, and especially in first-line medical services. I have wanted to indicate why this attitude is unjustified. I now proceed to discuss this in more detail, in connection with the phenomenon labeled 'patient paternalism'.

3. Paternalism

The practical difference between utilitarianism and deontology emerges in connection with paternalism. To act paternalistically, it will be assumed here, is to act in a certain way towards a person, even though the person has not asked for that particular action to be performed. If one acts paternalistically, one decides what is best for a person even though the person has not endorsed that action.

There are three kinds of patient paternalism that fall under this general definition (Wulff et al. 1990). The first is *genuine paternalism*. This kind of paternalism is applied when a patient is unable to choose what he wants to do (e.g. an unconscious person) or obviously lacks the capacity to know what is best for him (like a small child). Genuine paternalism is justified both according to utilitarianism and deontology. According to deontology, health workers should accept the choices only of an *autonomous* patient who knows what his best interests are.

The point is that if a patient who does not want necessary treatment is a small child or a person heavily influenced by drugs or alcohol, then he is not autonomous. In such cases both utilitarianism and deontology recommend that judgments about consequences should outweigh the patient's expressed wishes. That is, both positions imply that paramedics should choose the actions that they think have the best consequences for the patient. *Case 1* above appears to be a case of this kind. The reason is that the patient is agitated and stressed. He needs to calm down in order to properly understand the gravity of the situation and the potential negative consequences of his own expressed preferences.

The second form of patient paternalism is *desired paternalism*. This kind of paternalism is relevant when a patient wants someone else to decide what is best for him because he does not think he has the competence to decide himself. Suppose a paramedic is in the following situation:

> *Case 2* You are uncertain whether your patient should be transported to hospital or not. You ask the patient what he desires. The patient is informed about his condition and the different possibilities, but it is difficult for him to understand all the complex and detailed information you have given him. He says that he wants you to decide because he thinks you are more competent to make the correct decision.

As this case illustrates, desired paternalism often happens when a patient thinks a paramedic has more relevant medical knowledge than what he has himself. If the patient genuinely wants the paramedic to decide, then this is acceptable according to Kantian deontology. The reason is that the patient has freely chosen to leave the decision in the hands of the paramedic. One should then, as utilitarianism also recommends, choose the action that one thinks has the best consequences for the patient's health. Again, there is no conflict between utilitarianism and deontology. Both positions accept desired paternalism.

The conflict between utilitarianism and deontology arises in connection with the third and most extreme form of paternalism, *undesired paternalism*. To act paternalistically in this way is to refuse to let a patient do what he desires to do even though his preference is based on *autonomous* reasoning. In other words, the label 'undesired paternalism' can possibly apply only if the patient is autonomous (if the patient is not autonomous, then he is in the first category *genuine paternalism*).

Utilitarianism and deontology apparently advocate different actions in such situations: according to utilitarianism, it can be ethically correct to overrule the opinion of the patient if doing so is conceived to have the best consequences for him. In such cases, what the paramedic conceives to be best for the patient does not correspond to the patient's autonomous preferences. According to deontology, on the other hand, a paramedic must accept the preferences of an autonomous patient even if the paramedic thinks that these preferences do not have the best consequences for the patient's health.

I believe that this conflict between utilitarianism and deontology in connection with undesired paternalism corresponds to a fundamental question many paramedics have asked themselves: 'Should I do what I think has the best consequences for the patient, or should I do as the patient wishes that I do?' The two ethical positions give a more precise and explicit content to this experienced dilemma. I have shown that the main reason why the dilemma is experienced as a dilemma is that the conflicting considerations about the 'best' consequences and the patient's wishes correspond to a deep tension between utilitarianism and Kantian deontology.

4. Solving the problem

In many cases there is an *apparent* conflict between utilitarianism and deontology in connection with paternalism. Why make this reservation? Remember the above definition of deontology. According to the definition, a health worker should do as a patient wishes only if the patient is autonomous, if the action he endorses best serves his interests. So what if the patient is no longer in a state such that he is capable of free, rational reasoning? Or what if it is far from clear that the action he desires promotes his own, overall interests?

More generally, a deontologist holds that undesired paternalism can be justified if one of two conditions is met:

(1) The patient is not autonomous in the encounter with the paramedic.

(2) The patient will later come to realize that the course of action suggested by the paramedic best served his own interests.

If (1) or (2) is met, the conflict between utilitarianism and deontology makes no practical difference since both positions recommend paternalism if acting paternalistically is conceived to have the best consequences for the patient. According to deontology, it is acceptable to overrule the patient's own wishes and do what one thinks has the best consequences for him, if the patient's autonomy is impaired so that the situation involves genuine paternalism.

Of course, in some cases none of the conditions appear to be met. One example could be the following:

> *Case 3* A person has symptoms of having a fractured bone in his wrist. He is in pain but not to a very large extent, and he seems to be fully aware of the situation. You recommend transport to the hospital, so that the arm can be more fully examined. The person tells you that he will arrange with his own transport in 'half an hour' because there is something 'he has to do'.

In this case neither (1) or (2) seem to be met. Although the patient experiences some pain, he seems to be autonomous; his injury has not affected his ability to reason rationally and act in accordance with his own interests and knowledge of the consequences of his preference. There can therefore be a genuine conflict between utilitarianism and deontology, and in that case there is no straightforward solution to the dilemma: a paramedic who has strong consequence-based intuitions and thinks that the best consequences for the patient is to be transported right away will think that it is ethically correct to overrule the patient's expressed desire. A paramedic who has strong deontological intuitions will think that it is ethically correct to act in accordance with the patient's wishes.

However, although there are cases where it is far from clear that (1) or (2) are met, there appears to be very many cases where the conditions are met. Condition (1) is typically met when a person is in severe pain so that he has lost the capacity to reason rationally, or if he is in a special psychological state such as depression, anxiety or even panic. Patients (or relatives of patients) might also be in extreme emotional states such as shock and personal crises, due to an experience of sudden and dramatic loss of health (Nordby and Nøhr 2008; Nordby and Nøhr 2009). In such cases it is often reasonable to assume that the patient is no longer capable of autonomous reasoning, that he is not capable of acting freely in accordance with rational reasoning and his own overall beliefs and preferences.

The other condition (2) is met in cases when the patient will later come to realize that what the paramedic did best corresponded to what he 'really' wanted. *Case 1* above appears to be one such case: if the patient is not given treatment and transport, the probability of serious negative consequences is high. There is good reason to suppose that if the patient is given treatment in this case, he will later, when he has calmed down, agree that it was correct to do so. More generally, a deontologist will hold that paternalism is justified if a paramedic has good reason to suppose that the patient will later think that what the paramedic did best served his overall interests, including such wide issues as the patient's comprehensive perspective on himself, his family and the world around him.

A final example that illustrates this point even more clearly, is this:

> *Case 4* A person who is at a party and seems to be drunk has apparently received a brain concussion (and possibly a more serious head injury) from falling down from a balcony on the first floor. He claims that he is now 'feeling fine', and despite your detailed explanations, he insists on continuing the party.

In this case both (1) and (2) seem to be met. Condition (1) seems to be met because the person is apparently drunk and apparently not able to reason rationally and make free, independent choices. Condition (2) seems to be met because it is reasonable to assume that the person will later, when he is sober, agree that it was correct to give him necessary medical treatment.

The qualification 'seems to me met' is important. Perhaps the person is not really drunk even though it seems so? Furthermore, there is no guarantee that the person will later agree that it was correct to set aside his wishes. However, the point is that paramedics have to *act*. And if the choice is between an action that can have very serious negative consequences for the patient (in this case letting the patient decide), and an action that avoids dramatic negative consequences as well as possible, then it is better to be on the safe side.

In other words, as long as there is *good reason* to believe that a patient is not autonomous, then it is ethically correct to let the patient be transported and receive treatment as soon as possible, if this can prevent serious loss of health. One might even make stronger claim: unless it becomes evident that a patient is autonomous, the patient should be given necessary treatment as soon as possible if this can prevent dramatic negative consequences for him.

A paramedic should not, for the same reason, assume that a patient is autonomous unless he has very good reasons for assuming so. Again, this is especially important if letting the patient decide has dramatic consequences for the patient, and if the paramedic has strong 'deontological' intuitions in the sense explained above. In *case 3* above involving the fractured bone this was not crucial, since the negative consequences of letting the patient decide were not very serious. But in many other cases letting the patient decide can have dramatic consequences for the patient, and in these cases it must always be a good question if the patient has understood the gravity of the situation sufficiently well. In fact, within the limits of first-line medical emergency situations, it is extremely difficult to make sure that a patient is autonomous.

Further examples could be discussed, but doing so would fall outside the limits here. Determining the practical application of conditions (1) and (2) must also, I believe, be a job for paramedics themselves. What I have aimed to do is to develop some philosophical distinctions that I think can be useful in real life. As emphasized, it would be wrong to think that paramedics need certainty before they act on the basis of these distinctions. Fundamentally, if a paramedic has good reason to think that (1) or (2) is met, and if accepting the patient's expressed preferences has serious negative consequences for the patient, then the paramedic is, from an ethical point of view, justified in setting aside the patient's expressed wishes and instead do what he thinks is best for the patient.

5. Conclusion

Paramedics sometimes face an ethical dilemma: 'Should I do as the patient wishes that I do, or should I do what I think has the best consequences for the patient's health?' I have argued that this problem has a practical ethical solution in some important cases. In these cases it is reasonable to assume that the patient (1) does not have, or has temporarily lost, a capacity for rational reasoning or (2) will later come to realize that his expressed wishes did not best serve his own, overall interests. In such cases paternalism, doing what one thinks best prevents serious negative consequences related to the patient's health, is justified ethically, both according to utilitarianism and deontology. The difference between the ethical theories makes no practical difference.

As already indicated, I believe that paramedics have a pretheoretical understanding of the dilemmas surrounding paternalism and the distinction between utilitarianism and Kantian deontology. In this sense the aim of my discussion has not been to say something that is entirely new to paramedics. The idea has rather been to clarify and systematize intuitions paramedics already have. By being more aware of what the two ethical positions utilitarianism and deontology involve, it is easier for paramedics to know when paternalism is justified.

References

Befring A and Ohnstad B (2001). *Helsepersonelloven – med kommentarer.* Bergen: Fagbokforlaget 2001.

Clarke P and Linzey A (1996). *Dictionary of ethics, theology and society.* London: Routledge.

Harman G (1977). *The nature of morality: An introduction to ethics.* Oxford: Oxford University Press.

Kant I (1996). *The metaphysics of morals. Cambridge texts in the history of philosophy.* Cambridge: Cambridge University Press.

McKenna K and Sanders M (2001). *Workbook to accompany Mosby's paramedic textbook.* St. Lois/London: Mosby.

Mill J (1978). *On liberty.* Indianapolis: Hackett.

Nordby H and Nøhr Ø (2008). 'Communication in an emergency setting'. *Scandinavian journal of trauma, resuscitation and emergency medicine* 16, 5–10.

Nordby H and Nøhr Ø (2009). 'Interactive emergency communication with persons in crisis'. Forthcoming in *Journal of telecare and telemedicine.*

Ohnstad B (2002). *Rettigheter og plikter etter ny helselovgivning.* Bergen: Fagbokforlaget.

Sanders M (2001). *Mosby's paramedic textbook.* St. Louis/London: Mosby.

Wulff H, Pedersen S and Rosenberg R (1990). *Philosophy of medicine: An introduction.* Oxford: Blackwell.

Index

Index

Index